# CAN'T LIVE WITHOUT IT:
# THE STORY OF HEMOGLOBIN IN SICKNESS AND IN HEALTH

# CAN'T LIVE WITHOUT IT:
# THE STORY OF HEMOGLOBIN IN SICKNESS AND IN HEALTH

LOREN HAZELWOOD

**Nova Science Publishers, Inc.**
*Huntington, NY*

**Senior Editors:** Susan Boriotti and Donna Dennis
**Office Manager:** Annette Hellinger
**Graphics:** Wanda Serrano and Dorothy Marczak
**Information Editor:** Tatiana Shohov
**Book Production:** Cathy DeGregory, Jennifer Vogt and Lynette Van Helden
**Circulation:** Ave Maria Gonzalez, Mike Hedges, Ron Hedges and Andre Tillman

*Library of Congress Cataloging-in-Publication Data*

Hazelwood, Loren F.
  Can't live without it: the story of hemoglobin in sickness and in health / Loren Hazelwood.
    p. cm.
  Includes bibliographical references and index.
  ISBN 1-56072-907-4.
    1. Hemoglobin--Popular works. 2. Hemoglobinopathy--Popular works. 3. Anemia
  Popular Works. I. Title

  QP96.5 .H39 2001
  612.1'111--dc21

                                                                    2001030349

Copyright © 2001 by Nova Science Publishers, Inc.
              227 Main Street, Suite 100
              Huntington, New York 11743
              Tele. 631-424-6682        Fax 631-425-5933
              e-mail: Novascience@earthlink.net
              Web Site: http://www.nexusworld.com/nova

*Printed in the United States of America*

*For Donna*

# CONTENTS:

List of Figures and Tables ...........................................................................ix
Disclaimer ....................................................................................................xi
Preface ........................................................................................................ xiii
Acknowledgements ....................................................................................xvii
From Proteins to Politics ............................................................................. 1
The Search for Function ...............................................................................21
The Search for Structure...............................................................................39
Hemoglobin at Work ....................................................................................55
The Making of Hemoglobin ........................................................................71
Anemia ........................................................................................................85
Anemias of the Sea.......................................................................................93
The Major Genetic Variants .......................................................................103
Diabetes and Hemoglobin ..........................................................................117
Werewolves, Lead Poisoning, and King George III....................................129
Hemoglobin, Genetics and Public Policies ................................................139
A Short Review ...........................................................................................147
Glossary of Uncommon Words and Acronyms............................................157
Additional Readings ...................................................................................161

# LIST OF FIGURES AND TABLES

Figure 1. The Sickle ................................................................5
Figure 2. Normal and Sickled Red Cells. ..............................6
Figure 3. Basic Electrophoresis ..........................................13
Figure 4. Separation of Hemoglobins by Electrophoresis ............14
Figure 5. The Genetics of Sickle-Cell Anemia ....................15
Figure 6. Basic Pattern for Blood Circulation ....................21
Figure 7. Diagram of the Circulatory System ......................22
Figure 8. The Spectra of Hemoglobin ................................34
Figure 9. The Hüfner and Bohr Curves ..............................35
Figure 10. Measurement of Osmotic Pressure ....................40
Figure 11. Pyrolle ..............................................................42
Figure 12. Porphyrin ..........................................................43
Figure 13. Heme and Chlorophyll ......................................43
Figure 14. An Amino Acid ..................................................44
Table I: The Amino Acids in Hemoglobin ..........................45
Figure 15. Amino Acid Sequence of Alpha Chains ..............46
Figure 16. The Amino Acid Sequence of BetA Chains ........47
Figure 17. One Heme-globin Unit ......................................48
Figure 18. The Hemoglobin Molecule ................................49
Figure 19. Salt Bridges Between Globin Chains ..................51
Figure 20. Movement of the Heme Plane ............................52
Figure 21. Red Blood Cells of Vertebrates ........................57
Figure 22. The Respiratory System ....................................58
Figure 23. The Alveolus ....................................................58

Figure 24. Shifts in the Bohr Curve ................................................64

Figure 25. Red Blood Cell Production ............................................72

Figure 26. Structure of DNA ..........................................................74

Figure 27. Transfer RNA ................................................................75

Figure 28. The Synthesis of a Protein ............................................77

Figure 29. The Production of Heme ................................................79

Figure 30. Human Globin Chains ...................................................82

Figure 31. The Hematocrit .............................................................86

Table II. Normal Hemoglobin Levels .............................................87

Figure 32. Chromosome 11 ............................................................97

Figure 33. Chromosome 16 ..........................................................100

Figure 34. The Formation of Hb S Crystals ..................................107

Figure 35. Chromsome 11 Before Normal Meiosis .......................114

Figure 36. Formation of Hb Lepore and Anti-Lepore ...................115

Figure 37. Daily Blood Glucose Changes .....................................120

Figure 38. Changes in Hb $A_1$ Fractions ......................................125

# DISCLAIMER

This book is not intended to be medically authoritative. While every effort has been made to insure the information contained here is accurate, the reader should not rely on it for diagnosis of any health condition. Anyone believing they have a medical problem related to the topics covered in this book should seek the advice of a qualified physician.

# PREFACE

It was my original intention to use *Hemoglobin* as the title of this book, but several people advised against it. Although this single word seemed like the most natural summary of the subjects covered here, I was told that such a title, employing such a long and unfamiliar word, would imply to the prospective reader a highly technical medical text full of many strange, multi-syllabic words. This implication would, in turn, scare average people and keep them from even attempting to read the book. If true, this would have been very unfortunate. That is the very audience for whom I wrote this.

It is very important to make clear at the beginning that this is a popular science book. It is intended for any serious readers interested in learning more about how their bodies work and the role this one molecule has in their health. One does not need to have a background in biochemistry to understand the ideas presented here. For over 20 years I have been involved in the study and analysis of hemoglobin. During that period I have had to discuss the material in this book with people from a wide variety of backgrounds: physicians, research scientists, sales representatives, investment bankers, accountants, and interested people from the general public. Some had advanced college degrees; others had only a high school education. From my experiences I came to realize that people are interested in these subjects and are willing to learn the basic concepts when they are presented in the proper sequence to the appropriate level of details. In fact, a book on hemoglobin can serve as a platform from which the nonscientist can gain insights into the very basic concepts dealing with genetics, health, respiration, and several very important disease conditions. No one can live without hemoglobin, and millions of people in the world suffer from disorders related to the production and functioning of this one molecule.

Even if I could get people to open the book and not give up at the title, many were still skeptical that the average person could understand the material. But, I refuse to believe this is true. It has been my experience that the concepts presented here can be understood by anyone with "average" intelligence. The most important factors are motivation and patience. If these ideas can be understood by me, they can probably be understood by anyone interested enough to pick up this book and read it. My challenge has been to select the right material to discuss and to present it in the best sequence with the appropriate level of detail to make the ideas understandable. The readers' challenge is to have an open mind, to concentrate on the material, to review new ideas when necessary, and to have confidence in their own abilities to learn.

The idea of preparing this book came to me in 1982 when I was working on a small book describing a laboratory test that had been developed to monitor the care of diabetics*. (Don't bother to read it! The information that book contains has been updated here.) In the "Suggested Readings" section of that book I wrote that there was nothing available for the general reader on the hemoglobin molecule. What few books there were had been written for the specialist with a solid understanding of medicine or biochemistry, or both. There were no books that presented the subject in a "popular science" format. That observation motivated me to start this work, which will, I hope, satisfy that need.

I have tried to blend together chemistry, medicine, history, politics, and public health issues to approach the study of hemoglobin in as many ways as possible. No matter how basic I tried to make the material, there are some sections, especially those on respiration and genetics, that will, I know, be difficult for those readers who have a limited background in the sciences. I can only encourage them by saying that I have not introduced new concepts without presenting the basic principles needed to understand them. In many cases I have intentionally repeated information in order to help the reader review, assimilate, and understand new ideas. Before this book was published it was evaluated for me by a wide variety of people: high school graduates, college graduates with degrees not in the sciences, scientists, and physicians.

---

* The GHb Test, Loren Hazelwood. Charles Thomas, Publishers. Springfield, IL. 1982

For some the information in this book was a review; for others it was almost all new. They were all able to read the entire work, although some admitted to skimming lightly over Chapter 4 (on respiration) and Chapter 5 (on genetics). I encourage anyone reading this book who feels overwhelmed by the material at any point to move ahead rather than give up.

I also encourage everyone to read the chapters in the order presented, from start to finish. Much of what is discussed in each chapter is based on material previously covered. In addition, readers should look carefully at the illustrations when they are being discussed in the text. The figures are critical to understanding the material.

At the suggestion of my earliest reviewers I have added a Glossary at the end of the book with the pronunciation of some uncommon words and the definitions of some of the less common words and acronyms. If the word is not here, it will probably be found in any good dictionary.

Anyone who wishes to learn more about any of the topics in this book will find recommendations in the Additional Readings. Included are both very technical books and those suitable for the general reader.

Hemoglobin is an interesting molecule extremely important to the health of every human. The better we understand it, the more fascinating it becomes.

Enjoy the adventure.

*Loren Hazelwood*

# ACKNOWLEDGEMENTS

This book was <u>not</u> written with the financial support of any trust, fund, university, or government agency. But, it would have never been completed without the help of my friends and family. Many people volunteered to be readers of my first drafts, and I thank them for their suggestions, comments, and encouragement: Cecilia Getz, Bette Gualtieri, Kristen Chapman, Janine O'Neil, Lisa Gray, Andy Jaffe, Jan Brownlee, Janet Perkins, Barbara Baker, Helen Kuhar, Anita Kassuba and Amy Thackeray. Thanks also to Phyllis Komerofsky for typing my earliest efforts, before I bought my own computer.

I especially appreciate the support I have received from my wife, Donna, and my daughter, Jennifer.

*Chapter 1*

# FROM PROTEINS TO POLITICS

By any standard of measure hemoglobin is the most important protein in the human body.

In a normal day of healthy life the cells and tissues of the average adult manufacture thousands of proteins. More hemoglobin is produced than any other substance. Hemoglobin is found primarily in the red cells that circulate in the blood. These red cells are, in fact, little more than bags of a watery solution of hemoglobin molecules. Each particular hemoglobin molecule is created, does its work, and spends its entire life in one cell. Every healthy red cell lives for 120 days before it is destroyed. When that happens, the hemoglobin in it is also destroyed. Each *second* the body makes approximately seven million billion molecules of new hemoglobin to replace an equal number of old that have been destroyed during that same period. If there is a shortage of the raw materials available to make the molecules it needs, the body will give preference to the manufacture of hemoglobin.

To understand and appreciate the role of hemoglobin, it is helpful to remember that the human body is essentially a biological factory. It uses raw materials and energy to make products. Hemoglobin is one of those products, and its job is to deliver one of the raw materials needed for energy at each of the many work sites in the body.

The operating instructions for this factory are found in the genes.

We each started life as a single cell formed by the union of the genetic material from one mother and one father. That single cell contained two sets of instructions, one maternal and one paternal, for the manufacture of a large number of proteins. These proteins are essentially long chains of amino acids joined together. Drawing from a pool of 20 different amino acids, the body makes proteins by following the genetic information that dictates the exact sequence of amino acids to be used in the manufacture of each protein. From the beginning of life to the moment of death the body's cells continually follow these instructions to produce the proteins required for living. Some proteins are manufactured for a short period as needed to help the original cell grow and divide until it becomes an embryo, then a fetus, then a baby, then a mature adult. Other proteins help the body think, move, communicate, reproduce, and digest food. Hemoglobin itself serves to carry oxygen from the lungs to all the cells of the body and then returns with the waste carbon dioxide produced during the metabolism of food.

Those compounds of the body that are not proteins are either made by proteins or must be acquired in the diet. Steroids, for example, are not proteins. There is no genetic information about making a steroid directly. Instead, the cells must produce a specific set of proteins, and each protein is there to participate in a specific chemical reaction that is part of a series of reactions that result in the formation of a steroid. On the other hand, minerals like iron and calcium, many vitamins, carbohydrates, and eight of the amino acids needed to manufacture proteins cannot be made by the body. They must be obtained in the diet.

While the hemoglobin molecule is called a protein, its structure is more complicated than most proteins. One hemoglobin molecule contains four separate, but loosely bound segments — each a partnership of one globin and one heme. While the globin is a protein, the heme is not. Heme is a flat, disc-shaped molecule with space in the center for an iron atom. Thus, each hemoglobin molecule consists of four proteins, four non-proteins, and four iron atoms.

Since hemoglobin is the most important protein in the human body, it is not surprising that it is also the most studied. Recent studies of the complete human genetic code indicate that each person has the ability to manufacture approximately 30,000 different proteins. Hemoglobin is only one protein out of this number, yet more is known about it than any other. Scientists have been studying hemoglobin for over 150 years. In the last 30 years in particular there has been a tremendous amount of research on it. There is even one scientific journal that contains only articles about hemoglobin.

Why so much interest in this one protein? As we explore in this book the nature of hemoglobin and its function in the human body, it will quickly become obvious that this protein plays an extremely critical role in the health of each individual. We shall see that the continuous manufacture and proper functioning of hemoglobin are necessary to keep us alive, and problems with the hemoglobin molecule result in varying degrees of sickness for millions of people.

The initial scientific interest in hemoglobin was due to its role in transporting oxygen. Each milliliter[†] of normal, adult blood contains five billion red cells, and each of these red cells has approximately 300 million molecules of hemoglobin. It is, in fact, the hemoglobin that gives the cells, and the blood, their red color. Each one of these hemoglobin molecules can pick up four oxygen molecules in the lungs and carry them out to the cells and tissues of the body. Without oxygen these cells would die in a few minutes. The hemoglobin then helps carry the waste carbon dioxide produced in the cells back to the lungs. This process of respiration is extremely critical to the survival of the body, and hemoglobin has a unique structure that makes it particularly well suited to perform this task.

While we often speak of it as if it were a single substance, there are actually over 700 variants of the hemoglobin molecule. Some are normal components of the human body; others are genetic abnormalities. For example, the major hemoglobin component in fetal blood is not the same as that in the mother. The developing fetus must obtain oxygen from the maternal blood. Yet, there would be no reason for the mother's blood to give up oxygen to the fetus if the fetus' hemoglobin did not have a greater affinity for oxygen than the maternal. The normal adult hemoglobin, Hb[††] A, and the normal fetal hemoglobin, Hb F, are both considered normal hemoglobin components. They both occur naturally during the life of the majority of the members of the human race. The embryo, the fetus, and the adult each have their own normal hemoglobin components – all produced from information carried in the genetic code. There are only slight differences between these hemoglobin components, but these slight differences are critical for survival at each stage of life.

---

[†] Five milliliters (mL) is equal in volume to one teaspoon.
[††] Hb is a frequently used, but unofficial, abbreviation for hemoglobin.

There are also variants of the hemoglobin molecule that are the result of abnormal information in the genetic code. Some of these variants have no effect on the health of the individuals; others are so serious that they cause much pain and suffering – sometimes even an early death. Millions of people from China, southeast Asia, India, and Africa carry genes that produce abnormal hemoglobin molecules. Although the frequency is small, even northern Europeans can carry genes for abnormal hemoglobins.

In addition, there are genetic disorders in which the body produces reduced quantities of normal hemoglobin. Again, these disorders can range from very mild to extremely debilitating. Millions of people in the United States alone have some type of disorder related to the production of hemoglobin by the body. There is no gender, no age, and no ethnic background that escapes the potential for inherited or acquired disorders related to hemoglobin. People whose ancestors came from the Mediterranean region (Italy, Spain, Sicily, Greece, Turkey, the Middle East, and North Africa) have a high probability of carrying a gene that results in the underproduction of hemoglobin.

Iron-deficiency anemia, the most common nutritional disease in the world today, has as its major symptom decreased levels of hemoglobin in the blood.

Finally, there are molecules in the blood that are formed by a naturally occurring reaction between hemoglobin and glucose, a sugar. If the amount of glucose in the blood increases, more will react with hemoglobin to form these *glycohemoglobins*. The concentration of glycohemoglobins in the blood reflects how well the body can control its glucose levels. Someone whose blood glucose is higher than normal will have higher than normal amounts of glycohemoglobins. Even though diabetes is an endocrine disorder and has nothing to do with hemoglobin, it is possible to monitor its progress and treatment by measuring glycohemoglobins. This is important to the health of the millions of people in the world who have diabetes.

The diagnosis and treatment of the many forms of anemia, the mechanisms of lead poisoning, legends about werewolves, the causes of the American revolution, and the reelection of Richard Nixon are all issues related to the hemoglobin molecule. This substance is so important that there are programs in every state in the U.S., and in many other countries, to test the hemoglobin of every newly born child. These public health policies have raised serious questions about genetic counseling, treatment of genetic diseases, and prenatal screening.

Thus, in addition to its crucial role in respiration, hemoglobin is implicated in some of the most common genetic and nutritional diseases in humans and, hence, is associated with many serious public health issues. Disorders related to hemoglobin have affected our health, our history, our myths, our social structures, and our politics. This one protein is so important to us that it is little wonder it has attracted so much attention. While scientists have been studying hemoglobin since it was first isolated in the 1850's, the real interest in hemoglobin research was mainly the result of the discovery that a small variation in the hemoglobin molecule is responsible for sickle-cell anemia. Because this disorder has played such an important role in hemoglobin research, it is fitting to begin a discussion of hemoglobin by looking at sickle-cell anemia and its history.

There is little doubt that sickle-cell anemia has been around for thousands of years and has affected the lives of millions of people. Yet, it was not recognized by the medical community until this century. Dr. James Herrick, a Chicago physician, is credited with publishing the first description of a patient with sickle-cell anemia. In 1904 a young black student from the West Indies visited Dr. Herrick's office. The young man complained primarily of pains in his joints. He displayed the typical symptoms of anemia —— a general term given to many disorders where the patient lacks energy because of decreased production of red cells in the blood. When he looked at his patient's blood under a microscope, Dr. Herrick found two types of red cells. He found the normal, biconcave cells that look like a doughnut with a membrane pulled across the hole. But he also saw some red cells with a curved, elongated shape. They looked like a sickle, a tool with a long, curved blade attached to a short handle used to cut tall grasses and grains.

**Figure 1. The Sickle**

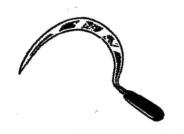

Dr. Herrick described his unusual patient in a talk given in 1905, and he later published a short report on the case in 1910[1]. There was little interest in the disease, however, and it was thought to be very rare. Only three additional cases had been reported by 1922 when Verne Mason described the same disorder in a patient at the Johns Hopkins Hospital. He wrote an article[2] on the case and gave the disease its name: sickle-cell anemia. The first part came from the fact that the presence of sickled cells in the blood distinguished this disorder from other types of anemia. It was called an anemia because that was the most common symptom of the disease.

It is important to remember that the symptoms of sickle-cell anemia are highly variable from person to person. There are bouts of pain in the joints — once or twice a year for some, 15-20 times a year for others. Some of these painful episodes are so serious they require hospitalization, treatment with painkillers, and intravenous administration of fluids. Sometimes clots form in the blood, resulting in a stroke or in damage to vital organs (heart, kidneys, lungs, liver or eyes). A clot near the skin may produce an ulcer, and clots in the lungs make the individual more prone to pneumonia or chronic lung disease. Many individuals with sickle-cell anemia have jaundice, which results in a yellowish appearance to their eyes. In addition, tiny blood vessels in the retina can be damaged, leading to problems with vision. Children with sickle-cell anemia often have problems with the growth and development of their bones. They also often have spleens so enlarged that they fill up the entire abdominal cavity.

**Figure 2. Normal and Sickled Red Cells.**

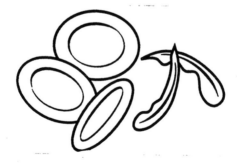

1 J. B. Herrick, "Peculiar elongated and sickle-shaped red corpuscles in a case of severe anemia," *Arch Int Med* 6:517, 1910.
2 Verne Mason, "Sickle cell anemia," *JAMA* 79:1318-1320, 1922.

The most common symptom is anemia. To be more specific, individuals with sickle-cell anemia often suffer from *hemolytic* anemia. The sickling of the red cells causes permanent damage to the cell membranes, and the cell can easily break apart, or hemolyze. There are then fewer cells to carry oxygen. Less oxygen to the cells means the body tires easily and often lacks the energy needed to perform normal tasks. The person with sickle-cell anemia must often avoid physical activities that, while they would represent little effort for some, will aggravate their condition and increase their pain.

Not every individual with sickle-cell anemia suffers all these problems to the same extent. The degree of severity varies. However, with such obvious symptoms, why did this disorder go unrecognized until 1904? Physicians had certainly seen people with sickle-cell anemia before but had given them some other diagnosis, such as general anemia, without recognizing the unique characteristics of the disorder. However, by the end of the nineteenth century the medical community was taking a serious interest in the chemical principles of medicine.

Dr. Herrick was not a general practitioner who just happened to notice unusual red cells in a patient's blood. At the age of 43 he took extra training in physical and organic chemistry while continuing his medical practice. He also traveled to Europe to study protein chemistry in the laboratory of Nobel-Prize winner Emil Fischer. Dr. Herrick was a careful clinical observer with a good chemistry background. In addition to being the first to recognize sickle-cell anemia, he was also the first person to describe the features of coronary thrombosis[3].

Dr. Herrick's method of detecting sickle-cell anemia by looking for sickled cells in a blood smear was further developed and refined into a standard laboratory technique by Victor Emmel. Dr. Emmel had grown up and worked on his father's farm in Kansas, and he had received little formal schooling before he was twenty. Then he decided to go to college and eventually earned a Ph.D. in anatomy at Brown University. In 1915 he was on the faculty at Washington University when the first person diagnosed with sickle-cell anemia was seen there.

Dr. Emmel's lab technique, which was to remain the standard method for diagnosing sickle-cell anemia for 30 years, involved placing a drop of blood

---

3 C. Lockard Conley, "Sickle-Cell Anemia - The First Molecular Disease," in *Blood, Pure and Eloquent*, M. M. Weintrobe (ed). New York: McGraw Hill, 1980.

between a sterile glass slide and a cover slip[4]. The edges of the cover slip were sealed with a petroleum jelly to keep out oxygen. The slide was then examined under a microscope to search for sickled cells.

Using this technique, investigators found that there are actually two different groups of people with red cells that can be made to sickle. Some people have blood filled with numerous sickled red cells. They generally have rather severe symptoms of the disorder. Others might have only an occasional sickled red cell but none of the other symptoms of sickle-cell anemia. Dr. Emmel found the red cells of the father of a patient with sickle-cell anemia could be made to sickle on the glass slide even though they were not found in his normal blood smear. The father displayed none of the symptoms seen in his child. It was assumed that these two situations represent different stages of development of the same disease. We now know that the father only carried the trait and his cells could only be made to sickle outside the body when placed in an abnormal environment depleted of oxygen.

Virgil Sydenstrucker, whose interest in sickle-cell anemia spanned over 30 years, was a professor at the Medical College of Georgia from 1922 to 1957. He carefully observed and recorded many of the symptoms of the disease and introduced the term "crisis" to describe the frequent bouts of pain encountered by those with sickle-cell anemia. He was also the first to observe that children with sickle-cell anemia are highly susceptible to infections and have a high mortality rate as a result of these infections. He originally believed that the "active" and "latent" stages of sickle-cell anemia are different phases of the same disorder[5].

Then, in 1933 L.W. Diggs demonstrated that there is a distinct difference between people with sickle-cell anemia and those who carry a slight sickling "trait" but have none of the other symptoms[6]. All the patients discovered thus far with sickle-cell anemia had been black, and it was assumed that it was a disease limited to the black race. Dr. Diggs studied over 3,000 black individuals and concluded that 8.3% of the black people in the United States possess the trait. He found that for every forty people who have the trait there is one person with sickle-cell anemia. In addition, Dr. Diggs developed the

---

4 V. E. Emmel, "A study of the erythrocytes in a case of severe anemia with elongated and sickle-shaped red blood corpuscles," *Arch Int Med* 20:586-598, 1917

5 C. Lockard Conley, *op. cit.*

6 L.W. Diggs, C.F. Ahmann and J. Bibb, "The incidence and significance of the sickle cell trait," *Ann Intern Med* 7:769-778, 1933.

first explanations as to why the sickled cells cause pain and anemia. He believed that the distorted shape of the cells prevented them from entering into and flowing smoothly through capillaries. These tiny blood vessels are so narrow that red cells can only pass through one at a time. In fact, the diameter of the capillaries is so small that each red cell must actually squeeze down to pass through. If the red cell is sickle shaped, it can plug the capillary and block the flow of blood. This blockage causes painful swelling and cuts off the flow of oxygen to that area of the body served by the blocked capillary.

In 1940 Irving Sherman[7] proved that in a person with sickle-cell anemia 30-60% of the red cells in the blood going to the heart (i.e., the venous blood) are sickled, but only 5-20% are deformed in blood leaving the heart (i.e., arterial blood). This indicates that the sickling of the cells is not an irreversible process. At least some of the cells that have been deformed can be returned to normal. This observation agreed with the report made by E. Vernon Hahn and Elizabeth Gillespie in 1927 that the sickling of the red cells occurs when the blood is low in oxygen[8]. Venous blood, containing less oxygen than arterial, will thus have a greater percentage of sickled cells. When blood receives oxygen in the lungs, some of the sickled cells resume their normal shape. It was also suggested at the time that sickling and unsickling could damage the cell membranes and decrease the life span of the cells. Later this was indeed proven to be the case.

While studies in the United States continued at a slow pace, doctors in West Africa began to report on cases of sickle-cell anemia in that region. In 1944 a study conducted there indicated that approximately 20% of the population carried the trait. So many in the area had died for other reasons that the extent of sickle-cell anemia had not been noticed before. The high levels of infant mortality, the lower standards of health care, poor nutrition, and the prevalence of infections had all helped to mask the presence of the disorder. Where health care improved the frequency of sickle-cell anemia became noticeable.

---

7 I. J. Sherman, "The sickling phenomenon, with special reference to the differentiation of sickle cell anemia with sickle cell trait," *Bull Johs Hopkins Hosp* 67:309-324, 1940.

8 E. V. Hahn and E. B. Gillespie, "Sickle cell anemia. Report on a case greatly improved by splenectomy. Experimental study of sickle cell formation," *Arch Int Med* 39:233-254, 1927.

By 1950 the medical community began to realize the extent of sickle-cell anemia in the world. In the U.S. about one out of ten blacks carries the trait. They suffer no adverse health effects but can pass this trait on to their children. In some regions of Africa up to 40% of the population carries the trait. It is also found in Sicily, southern Italy, Greece, Turkey, Arabia, and south India.

Although many think of sickle-cell anemia as a disease of the black race, this is not the case. It is also found in some whites of Mediterranean ancestry, in many people in the Arabian peninsula, and in several areas of India. Sickle-cell anemia does not appear to be related specifically to race as much as to the geographical origin of one's ancestors. In 1952 a physician in Southern Rhodesia wrote a letter[9] to the British Medical Journal suggesting that "red cells in sicklers offer a less favorable environment for malarial parasites." Malaria is caused by a protozoan parasite (*Plasmodium falciparum*) that spends part of its life cycle in humans and part in the anopheles mosquito. In humans with malaria this small, single-celled organism lives and reproduces primarily in red blood cells. Thus it would seem that a "defect" or variation in the red cell might in some way inhibit the development of the parasite. In 1954 A.C. Allison found that in areas where malaria is endemic people with sickle-cell trait suffer from malaria less frequently and less severely than those without the trait[10]. The pattern of distribution of areas of the world where sickle-cell anemia seems to have originated is similar to that of the malarial regions of the world before modern medicine. This has led some to believe that the sickle-cell gene has survived because carriers of the trait are more resistant to malaria than normal individuals. The modern reader, for whom malaria may seem to be a rare tropical disease, may not realize the implications of this connection. However, as one medical historian has pointed out:

> If we consider the impact of diseases on populations over time as measured by the greatest harm to the greatest number, malaria has been the most devastating disease in history[11].

---

9 P. Brain, "Sickle-cell anemia in Africa," *British Medical Journal* 2:880, 1952.

10 A.C. Allison, "Protection afforded by sickle-cell trait against subtertian malarial infection," *British Medical Journal* 1:290-294, 1954.

11 Lois N. Magner, *A History of Medicine*, Marcel Dekker, Inc., New York, 1992, pg. 223.

When invaded by the malarial parasite, normally stable red cells of someone with sickle-cell trait can sickle in a low oxygen environment (e.g., in the veins). The sickling process destroys the invading organism and prevents it from spreading through the body. This apparent ability of a genetic condition to protect carriers is particularly important in infants. Thus, in regions repeatedly devastated by malaria, people who carry the trait for sickle-cell anemia will have a greater chance for survival than normal individuals.

Many believe that the sickle-cell trait originated during the Neolithic Age in Arabia and then spread by migration eastward to India and westward to Africa. Certainly it has been spread even faster over the centuries by the transportation of Africans as slaves to the Persian Gulf, to India, and, most recently, to the Americas.

While the genetic character of sickle-cell anemia was well accepted by 1950, there was still a question as to what exactly causes the red cells to deform. How are the red cells of an individual with sickle-cell anemia different from those of a normal individual? Dr. Diggs had noticed that the red cells of newborns with sickle-cell anemia sickled more slowly and in smaller numbers than in an adult. In 1948 Janet Watson concluded that hemoglobin is probably the culprit[12]. The hemoglobin in a newborn is different from that in an adult. After birth the fetal hemoglobin (Hb F) is gradually replaced by adult Hb A. She felt that the problem was due to some alteration in the hemoglobin A. This would explain why there was little sickling in newborns (with high levels of F) and increased sickling in the blood as A replaces F.

In 1945 Dr. Linus Pauling, a chemist from the California Institute of Technology, met Dr. William Castle, a physician and professor of medicine at the Harvard Medical School. Dr. Castle was an expert in anemia and had discovered the cause of pernicious anemia. He had become interested in sickle-cell anemia in 1938 when a white woman of Italian descent was admitted to Boston City Hospital with the disease. Dr. Castle and Dr. Pauling had been appointed to a committee that was to make recommendations to the government about what it should do to promote medical research after World War II[13]. In the course of their conversations Dr. Castle described to Dr.

---

12 J. Watson, A.W. Stahman, and F.P. Bilello, "The significance of the paucity of sickle cells in newborn Negro infants," *Am J Med Sci* 215:419-423, 1948.
13 C. Lockard Conley, *op. cit.*

Pauling the research he was doing on sickle-cell anemia and the changes seen in the shape of the red cell. Not only did this happen in the body of an individual with the disease, he reported, but this same sickling phenomenon could be seen in a solution of the patient's blood from which oxygen had been removed. At the time most physicians felt that the sickling was due to a defect in the membrane that surrounds the red cell.

Dr. Castle's words fell on the ears of a man whose mind was prepared to receive the information and quickly jump to the correct conclusion. Linus Pauling had spent many years investigating the structures of molecules and the nature of the chemical bonds between atoms. In 1933 and 1936 he had studied hemoglobin and published a paper on its magnetic properties. He had continued to do research on the structure of proteins and was familiar with the crystalline properties of various human and animal hemoglobins. He knew that hemoglobins could be made to form long needle-like crystals under certain conditions. During the course of their discussions it occurred to Pauling that the hemoglobin in patients with sickle-cell anemia might be a genetic mutation — a hemoglobin molecule slightly different from the normal. He also envisioned that this particular mutation would result in a hemoglobin molecule of a different type that would easily crystallize in the absence of oxygen. These crystals would be long, like needles, and would grow so large that they would deform the cell's membrane[14].

After he returned to California, Dr. Pauling asked one of his students, Harvey Itano, an M.D. working on his Ph.D., to study the problem. Dr. Itano obtained blood samples from normal individuals, from patients with sickle-cell anemia, and from individuals with the trait. He and his colleague, S.J. Singer, compared the three samples using electrophoresis, a laboratory technique that separates molecules on the basis of their electrical charge in a solution. If there were any differences in the hemoglobins in the three samples, they might be separable by electrophoresis.

Today the separation of hemoglobin variants by electrophoresis is a relatively simple technique that can be done in a few minutes in most clinical laboratories. The electrophoresis equipment consists of two tanks with a strip of a solid material stretched between them. The solid material may be made from cellulose acetate (and look like a strip of paper) or consist of a thin layer

---

14 Linus Pauling, "Fifty years of progress in structural chemistry and molecular biology," *Daedalus* (1964), pp. 988-1014.

of agarose, a seaweed extract, on a plastic sheet. Electrodes are placed in each tank, and the tanks are filled with buffered solutions. An electrical circuit is formed that conducts current from one electrode, through a buffer, across the solid material, into the other tank of buffer, and finally into the second electrode. (See .) If a solution of hemoglobin is placed on the solid strip and a voltage applied to the electrode, the hemoglobin molecules will move toward the negative electrode. When the blood of a person with sickle-cell anemia is analyzed next to that of a normal individual, the hemoglobins are seen to migrate to different locations. The sickle-cell hemoglobin has a greater positive charge than normal hemoglobin and will move toward the negative electrode at a faster rate. The blood of a person with sickle-cell trait has two different hemoglobins: one moves like the normal molecule while the other migrates like the hemoglobin from a person with sickle-cell anemia. illustrates a side-by-side separation of the two hemoglobins from the three samples.

This procedure is now done routinely in less than an hour. At that time it was a new and relatively complex technique, and the work was not finished until 1949. While the complete structure of hemoglobin was not known, it had long been observed that the substance has two components. It contains a colorless protein and a colored material that is not a protein. I.C. Wells, a fourth member of Pauling's group, proved that the non-protein portions of the three samples were identical. This would imply that any differences in the hemoglobin molecules would be due to differences in the proteins. Since the structure of proteins is controlled by the genes, the differences had to be inherited. Their report was printed in *Science* in 1949[15].

## Figure 3. Basic Electrophoresis

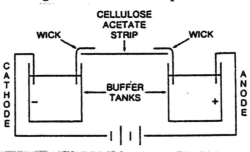

---

15 Linus Pauling, Harvey Itano, S.J. Singer, and Ibert C. Wells, "Sickle Cell Anemia, a Molecular Disease," *Science* 110: 543-548, 25 Nov 1949.

Pauling, Itano, Singer and Wells found that there were two different hemoglobins in their three samples. The hemoglobin of the normal individual was already labelled as Hb A. The patient with sickle-cell anemia had a different hemoglobin that they designated Hb S. The blood of the person with sickle-cell trait had a mixture of both A and S with slightly more A than S.

The implications of this study were tremendous. For the first time it was possible to point to a specific molecule in the body and say that it is responsible for a certain disease. The Hb S in people with sickle-cell anemia has properties slightly different from those of Hb A. These differences result in a molecule that can crystallize in a low oxygen environment more easily than Hb A, and it is this crystal formation that causes the sickling of the cells, the plugging of capillaries, and other symptoms of sickle-cell anemia. On the other hand, those who are only carriers of the trait have both A and S. The presence of A prevents the S from crystallizing under normal conditions, and there is little danger from sickling of cells. This also explains why newborns with sickle-cell anemia have few sickled cells until they are older. The Hb F prevents the S from sickling until F has disappeared and been replaced by S.

### Figure 4. Separation of Hemoglobins by Electrophoresis

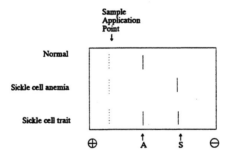

In 1949 James Van Neel at the University of Michigan, without knowing the molecular basis for the disease, published a proposed genetic pattern to describe the inheritance of sickle-cell anemia[16]. His results reinforced the work of Pauling's group and indicated that sickle-cell anemia is passed on from generation to generation in the genes. The laws of this inheritance are simple and straightforward.

---

16 J.V. Neel, "The inheritance of sickle cell anemia," *Science* 110:64-66, 1949.

**Figure 5. The Genetics of Sickle-Cell Anemia**

A. Why each child of two healthy parents has a 25% chance of inheriting sickle-cell anemia if both parents are carriers of the trait.

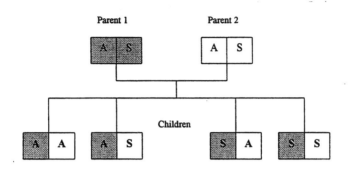

Each parent donates one of two genes. There are four equally likely combinations: AA, AS, SA, and SS. AS and SA are the same. Therefore, each child has a one in four (25%) chance of being AA; two chances out of four (50%) of being AS; and a one in four (25%) chance of being SS

B. The possible children of parents when only one carries the sickle-cell trait.

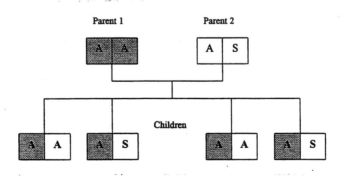

Each child has a 50% chance of inheriting the trait (AS) and a 50% chance of being AA. There is no possibility for SS.

C. The possible children of a person with sickle-cell anemia whose spouse is normal.

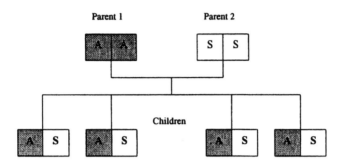

Every child will have a 100% chance of carrying the trait. None will have sickle-cell anemia.

D. The possible children of a person with sickle-cell anemia whose spouse has sickle-cell trait.

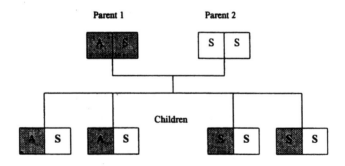

Each child has a 50% chance (two out of four) of being a carrier and a 50% chance of having sickle-cell anemia.

Each person receives from each parent a complete set of genes that tell the body how to make hemoglobin. The normal individual has two sets of Hb A genes and can be designated AA. If, on the other hand, one parent passes one S gene and the other provides an A, the child is AS. An AS person has received from one parent the genetic information needed to make normal, adult hemoglobin A but from the other the information that results in Hb S. Both are produced. Those who receive S genes from both parents are SS. They can make only hemoglobin S and have sickle-cell anemia.

This scheme explains how two healthy people can have a child with sickle-cell anemia. Assume both parents are carriers of the trait, i.e., they are AS. They will suffer no adverse health effects from carrying the trait, but they can each pass either an A or an S gene to each of their children. There are only three possible combinations of genes from AS parents. The children can be AA, AS or SS. The probability of AA or SS is 25% while that of AS is 50%. (See Figure 5A.) Each child born of these parents has a 25% chance of having sickle-cell anemia, a 50% chance of being a carrier of the trait, and a 25% chance of not having an abnormal gene at all.

It will also help to understand the genetics of sickle-cell anemia if we look at other possible situations. Assume that one parent is AA and the other is AS, then each child has a 25% chance of carrying the trait (AS) and a 75% chance of having no abnormal gene (AA). (Figure 5B.) If someone with sickle-cell anemia marries someone who is AA, all their children will be carriers of the trait but none will have the disease. (Figure 5C.) If, however, one spouse is SS and the other AS, then each child will have a 50% chance of having sickle-cell anemia and a 50% chance of being a carrier only. (Figure 5D.)

The next obvious question is how Hb S differs from Hb A. Since hemoglobin contains protein made from amino acids joined together, Pauling believed that S differed from A in the exact sequence of these amino acids. In 1955 Vernon Ingram in England found that S and A differ in only one out of 287 amino acids[17]. It is this single difference that changes the properties of hemoglobin and gives S its ability to so readily form crystals.

The idea that changes in proteins could be the result of variations in genes, while well understood today, was still unproven in the early 1950's. Once

17 V.M. Ingram, "A specific chemical difference between the globins of normal and sickle-cell anemia hemoglobin," *Nature* 178:792, 1956.

Watson and Crick had described the structure of DNA in 1953, the road was open for demonstrating how genetic information could be translated to the detailed manufacture of proteins by the body. The research by Pauling's group was the first to show that a mutant gene can result in a change in a single protein that is responsible for a specific disease condition.

For the next twenty years research in sickle-cell anemia proceeded at a slow but steady pace. There was a segment of the medical community interested in hemoglobin and actively studying its structure and variants. They were looking for a cure to sickle-cell anemia. Then, on February 18, 1971, President Nixon gave a speech to the Congress with his proposals for a national health strategy for the seventies. He singled out two specific diseases: cancer and sickle-cell anemia. For cancer, a disease known to everybody, the President proposed to expand the current research program by 100 million dollars. He increased the budget for sickle-cell anemia, a disease known to few, to a **total** of five million dollars.

Even before the President's speech there had been an increasing public interest in sickle-cell anemia. Much of this attention was due to the efforts of one man: Leonard Patricelli[18]. In November 1970 Mr. Patricelli, the President of WTIC television and radio in Hartford, CT, gave four prime time editorials on the subject. The station followed the editorials with four documentaries that generated interest throughout the state. This publicity and Mr. Patricelli's efforts led to the passage of sickle-cell legislation by the State of Connecticut (the first state to do so) and raised $40,000 to help start a Sickle-Cell Center at Howard University in Washington, D.C.

Mr. Patricelli had apparently learned about sickle-cell anemia from his son, Robert, at that time a deputy undersecretary at the Department of Health, Education and Welfare. HEW officials were preparing information for the President's health message, and the younger Patricelli received a report on sickle-cell anemia written by Colby King. The report was the result of a letter from a black woman who had written to HEW asking for help with her son, who had the disease.

Leonard Patricelli felt that it was time to bring the extent and nature of the disease to the attention of the public. His editorials anticipated President Nixon's speech by several months. Some believe that the President's primary

18 Barbara Culliton, "Sickle Cell Anemia: The Route from Obscurity to Prominence," *Science* 178:138-142, 13 Oct 1972.

motive was to attract more support and votes from the black community. Whatever the reasons, Nixon's speech and the Hartford T.V. programs were major factors in bringing sickle-cell anemia to the public's attention and making it a disease of national importance.

The Department of Health, Education, and Welfare originally asked for 5 million dollars: $2.5 million for the creation of no more than five comprehensive research and service centers, $1 million for screening clinics (between 10 and 20) and $1.5 million for research toward better treatment of sickle-cell anemia. But this was not enough for Congress. The upheaval of popular support created interest in the Congress, and the authorization was increased to $25 million for the 1973 fiscal year. This amount was to be further increased to $40 million in 1974 and $50 million in 1975. There were soon 250 centers in the U.S. distributing educational materials and screening for sickle-cell anemia. Naturally, some of this new funding went toward sponsoring research into the nature of the molecule that is the cause of the disease. President Nixon's political concerns led to an increase in research on hemoglobin and its variants.

Now the National Sickle-cell Disease Program is a permanent part of the Division of Blood Diseases and Resources of the National Heart, Lung and Blood Institute, one of the National Institutes of Health. The program supports basic research, clinical research, treatment trials, professional and paraprofessional education programs, public education, screening, counseling, and related activities.

The public attention given to sickle-cell anemia along with the widespread existence of other hemoglobin related disorders and the extremely important role of hemoglobin in body chemistry have all combined to make this one protein the most studied in the human body.

The story of sickle-cell anemia offers an excellent case study to introduce hemoglobin, but it is only a small part of the complete picture. The next two chapters will review the history of the development of our knowledge about the function and structure of hemoglobin. Chapter 4 will explain how hemoglobin works and the role it plays in respiration, and Chapter 5 will discuss the production of hemoglobin. Once it is clear how hemoglobin works in healthy individuals, it will be easier to appreciate how various illnesses are caused by inherited or acquired disorders related to the production of hemoglobin. These disorders will be discussed in Chapters 6, 7, 8, and 10. Chapter 9 will cover glycohemoglobins and how they can be used to help diabetics. Finally, in Chapter 11 we will return to the public health issues that continue to generate interest in hemoglobin.

Only by approaching this subject from so many different directions – historical, molecular, genetic, functional, physiological, and political – can one begin to understand this fascinating substance.

# Chapter 2

# THE SEARCH FOR FUNCTION

The quest for understanding the role of hemoglobin in the body really began with investigations into the nature and purpose of blood. For it is in the blood that the hemoglobin molecule performs its critical job of carrying oxygen to all the cells and tissues of the body. The red blood cells, which contain hemoglobin, form about one-half of the total volume of blood. The rest of the blood, the plasma, contains many other substances not related to gas transport. The blood stream has many roles in the body. It removes carbon dioxide, excess water, and other waste products and carries them to the lungs and kidneys for elimination. Nutrients reach the cells through the blood system. White cells are swept along with the blood while they await signs of infection by foreign materials or organisms. Platelets and a complex system of molecules float around waiting for a break in the walls of the blood vessels so they can form a clot to prevent the loss of blood. And hormones, chemical messengers from the endocrine glands, travel through the blood to reach their destinations.

**Figure 6. Basic Pattern for Blood Circulation**

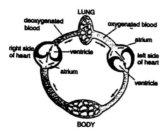

This fluid is so vital to the body's life that it must circulate continuously beginning a few weeks after conception; it does not stop until death. The blood flows through the body in two separate circuits. First, it goes to the lungs to be enriched with oxygen and then returned to the heart. This is the pulmonary circulation. It then is sent out to the all the tissues of the body and returned back to the heart to start the cycle over again. To keep the blood flowing in both these cycles requires the regular expansion and contraction of the heart muscle.

The heart consists of four chambers — two larger, called the left and right ventricles, and two smaller, the atria, located on top of the ventricles. From the right ventricle the heart pushes the blood into the lungs through the pulmonary artery. (An artery is any vessel that carries blood away from the heart; a vein carries it to the heart.) In the lungs hemoglobin picks up oxygen, and the blood returns enriched with oxygen to the left atrium of the heart via the pulmonary vein.

## Figure 7. Diagram of the Circulatory System

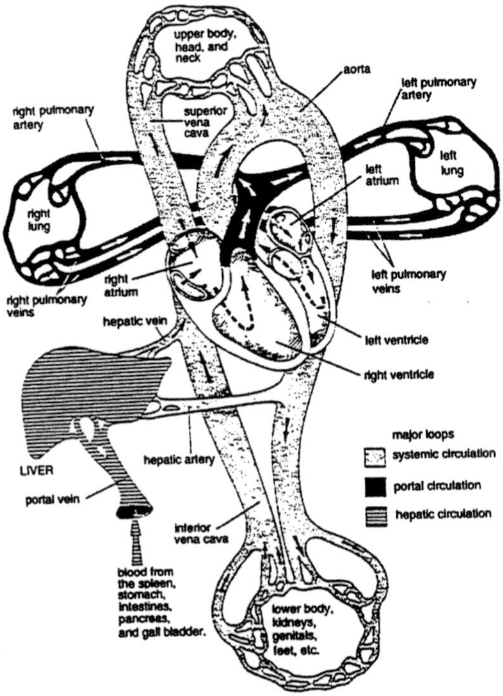

The blood then passes from the left atrium to the left ventricle. From there it is forced out into the aorta and on through the major arteries. These blood vessels have thicker walls than the veins and can withstand the pressures generated as the heart muscle pushes the blood through them. As the arterial system spreads through the body the vessels branch out, subdivide, and continue to split the blood into smaller and smaller streams. Finally, the blood must pass through a capillary — a vessel so narrow that only one red cell at a time can squeeze through. It is here in the capillaries that the blood comes closest to the body's cells and delivers oxygen and nutrients. At the same time waste products from the cells are picked up and swept away.

The small capillaries merge to form veins that join to create larger veins that finally return blood back to the right atrium of the heart. Because the pressure in the veins is lower and pulsates less than in the arteries, the veins do not need such thick walls. However, they do have small one-way valves located at regular intervals to prevent the back flow of blood into the heart. Blood from the lower part of the body and blood returning from the liver come to the right atrium in the inferior vena cava. Blood from the head and neck is returned in the superior vena cava. Blood from the two returning streams mixes in the right atrium and enters the right ventricle, where the circuit starts over again. In its travels the blood has also passed through the kidneys to allow for waste removal, taken oxygen and nutrients to the heart muscle so it can function, passed by endocrine glands to pick up any hormones being produced, and collected nutrients absorbed from the stomach and the intestines.

Blood is so essential to life and performs so many functions that it is not surprising that early cultures recognized its necessity even though they had no knowledge of its circulation or concept of its purpose. Some ancient philosophers thought it was the seat of consciousness and that we reason with our blood. Others believed its function was to cool the body, especially in the region around the heart. Many ancient people believed that the soul of an animal is in the blood. Hence the prohibition against the eating of blood given in Genesis and Leviticus, and the Jewish rituals for the slaughter of animals that prevent the mingling of blood with meat:

> But you must not eat the flesh with the life, which is the blood, still in it. (Genesis 9:4)

Any Israelite or alien settled in Israel who hunts beasts or birds that may
lawfully be eaten shall drain out the blood and cover it with earth, because
the life of every living creature is the blood, and I have forbidden the
Israelites to eat the blood of any creature, because the life of every creature is
its blood: every man who eats it shall be cut off. (Leviticus 17: 13-14)

It was also a common concept among early mankind to believe that
character traits of people reside in the blood and can be passed via the blood
from one generation to another. It is still part of our language to refer to
someone as possessing "good" or "bad" blood or to say that someone has
Indian or African or Jewish or Irish "blood" flowing in their veins. The
modern interpretation is that the person has inherited traits common to a
certain nation or race or behavior pattern, but the common language still
contains the ancient misconception that these qualities were carried in the
blood.

Early Greek medicine was based on the idea that an illness is caused by
unknowable supernatural forces. The earliest healers were priests who would
diagnose the causes and treatments of diseases on the basis of patients' dreams
and other oracular techniques. The followers of Hippocrates were the first
physicians to assume that there is a logic behind the universe and that it
operates by rational rules.

Hippocrates (b. 460 B.C. on the island of Cos, near the western coast of
Asia Minor) learned medical skills from his father and developed a reputation
as an excellent physician and great teacher. A collection of 70 scientific
treatises produced at the medical academy of Cos were ascribed to him.
Hippocrates was probably not the author of all the works, but the collection
has come down to us under his name. The philosophy of Hippocrates and his
followers encouraged the physician to make observations of the patient in an
attempt to deduce the natural causes of the disease. This was the earliest
experimental approach to understanding the human body and essentially
formed the basis for using scientific methods in medicine.

For the Hippocratic physician Nature desires to maintain stability and
equilibrium among the constituents of the body. When there is a balance, the
person is healthy. When, for some reason, the equilibrium is upset, sickness
develops. The function of the physician is to help Nature restore the body to
the state of equilibrium. Hippocrates taught that the primary constituents of

the body are four fluids, or humors: blood, yellow bile, black bile, and phlegm. Blood was thought to originate in the heart, yellow bile in the liver, black bile in the spleen, and phlegm in the brain. Illness was due to an imbalance of the four humors. The physician's work then is to look carefully at the symptoms of the patient to determine the excess of which humor was responsible for the disorder.

This approach to understanding the body has held on for so long that people were still being routinely bled in the eighteenth century to cure them of an excess of blood.

The early Greeks had little knowledge of actual anatomy. Most conclusions were based on the dissection of animals and occasional experiences with human bodies. However, the Hippocratic writings did recognize that there is a difference between arteries and veins. The veins contained blood, but the arteries were said to carry air. This conclusion probably came from observations that the arteries in a corpse are empty. At death the muscular contractions of arterial walls force blood into the capillaries and veins. Hence, dissection of the body of one who has died reveals two types of blood vessels: one with blood in them (veins) and one with air (arteries).

For a brief period during the third and fourth centuries B.C. learning in the sciences and engineering flourished in Alexandria in Egypt. There had been such a long history of embalming and preparing bodies for burial in Egypt that the people did not have any traditional opposition to dissection. Herophilis of Chalcedon (333-280 B.C.), who studied and taught for many years in Alexandria, is said to have been the first physician to dissect human bodies in public. Many consider him the founder of the science of anatomy. He recognized that the brain, and not the heart, is the seat of intelligence, and that both arteries and veins carry blood. He found that arteries have thicker walls than veins and recognized that the heart sends blood into the arteries.

Erasistratus of Chios (310-250 B.C.), a younger contemporary of Herophilis, also lived and worked at Alexandria. He taught that blood is the source of matter in the body and is carried by veins. He maintained that the air taken in by the lungs is changed to pneuma in the heart and sent to the various parts of the body through the arteries. He noted that if you cut the artery in a living body it would contain blood. He explained this by saying that the pneuma escaping from the artery creates a vacuum that draws in blood through very fine connections between the veins and the arteries. In other words, he guessed at the presence of capillaries. He recognized that the heart is a pump and deduced that the tricuspid valve (between the right atrium and the right ventricle), the bicuspid valve (between the left atrium and the left ventricle), and the semi-lunar valves (at the outlets of the ventricles) are all designed to allow material to pass in one direction only.

The development of the ancient concepts of blood and its function in the body reached its ultimate form in the writings of Galen, a Roman physician of the second century A.D. Born to Greek parents in Pergamum in 130 A.D., during the reign of the Emperor Hadrian, Galen began his study of medicine at age 15. He became physician to the gladiators in Pergamum at age 28. Since the dissection of human bodies was forbidden, Galen undoubtedly learned a great deal of his anatomy treating the wounds of the gladiators. Later he moved to Rome and gained such a reputation that he became the court physician first to Emperor Marcus Aurelius and then to his son, the Emperor Commodus. He is said to have produced 500 treatises in Greek on many subjects, but only 100 have survived.

According to Galen blood is manufactured in the liver out of 'chyle' from the intestines. It is then carried to all parts of the body by the veins, although the arteries are used to some extent. (He did state that the arteries carried blood and not air.) The blood, he claimed, is then carried to the left side of the heart where impurities are removed and transported to the lungs for elimination. In the heart the blood passes from the left side to the right through small holes in the septum (the muscular wall that divides the left and right ventricles). These holes were too small to be seen with the naked eye, but Galen knew they had to be there.

Galen's concept of blood flow was generally accepted by European and Islamic scientists for over 1,000 years. It is one of the great ironies in the history of science that although he himself believed strongly in the value of experience and experimentation, Galen's works became sacred texts to the medical profession. Teachers of anatomy put such faith in Galen that they would simply read his books to students while an assistant, when permitted by local laws and customs, dissected cadavers. In the fourteenth century the Italian professor of anatomy Mondino de'Luzzi (1275-1326) broke with that tradition and carried out dissection himself. He noted many details at variance with the statements of Galen and published these observations in his book in

1315. Unfortunately other professors did not follow his example and retained the older method. Jacobus Sylvius, a leading professor of anatomy in Paris in the late fifteenth century, shared the common view that if a dissected body differed from what Galen described, it must be because human anatomy had changed over the centuries. For 200 years there was no continuation of the advances made by Mondino, and the books of Galen continued to occupy a position of unquestioned authority.

Many of the inconsistencies between Galen's texts and actual human anatomy were due to Galen's need to rely on dissection of monkeys and pigs to form his conclusions. Roman, medieval European, and Islamic customs all forbade dissection of the human body. It wasn't until dissection became acceptable in the 15th and 16th centuries that anatomists seriously began to question Galen. They found too many inconsistencies and too many unanswered problems. They were particularly bothered by their inability to see or demonstrate the existence of the small pores that Galen assured them had to be in the wall between the two lower chambers of the heart.

Andreas Vesalius (1514-1564), the preeminent anatomist of the sixteenth century, was born and educated in Brussels. He became professor of surgery and anatomy at the University of Padua, the most esteemed medical school in Europe. In his teaching Vesalius did not follow the traditional practice of reading from a book while an assistant dissected a body for students. He lectured to the students who watched while he himself did the dissection.

In 1543 Vesalius published a seven-volume book with detailed anatomical drawings. His *De Humanis Corpis Fabrica* changed the course of research into human anatomy. He noted discrepancies between his observations and Galen's texts. He also proved that Galen had relied on the dissection of apes in his studies. However, he did not spot all Galen's errors. His diagrams still indicated perforations between the two ventricles of the heart.

In 1553 Michael Servetus, a Spanish physician, theologian, and former law student, published his book *De Christianismi Restitutione* (The restoration of Christianity) with comments on the Bible and his theories about the circulation of the blood. Servetus was a scholar with wide-ranging interests and strong independence of mind. His religious views were so controversial that he was persecuted by the Catholic Inquisition in France and burned at the stake by John Calvin in Geneva. He studied medicine in Paris and while there reached the conclusion that the blood is pumped from the right ventricle to the lungs, back to the heart, and then out to the body. This is the earliest description of pulmonary circulation in European literature.

There is no indication as to how Servetus reached this conclusion about the pulmonary circulation of the blood. It may have simply been the results of his careful observations as a medical student whose questioning mind refused to accept the standard "truths," whether medical or theological. However, twentieth century scholars have discovered that the existence of pulmonary circulation was known to a thirteenth century Egyptian doctor, Ibn al-Nofis[19]. An Islamic scientist and Chief of Physicians in Egypt, Ibn al-Nofis wrote books on a wide variety of topics (medicine, logic, law, ethics, languages, and rhetoric), but his works appear to have been largely ignored by the West until this century. In 1215 al-Nofis not only wrote the earliest description of pulmonary circulation, he also asserted that, contrary to the writings of Galen, there are no passages between the right and left ventricles that could permit blood to flow between the two chambers of the heart. The Islamic world also frowned on the dissection of bodies, so we are not certain what led him to arrive at these conclusions. Even though he was not widely known in European science, it does appear that a Latin translation of the works of Ibn al-Nofis was published in Venice in 1547. Servetus may have known the work, or he may have independently observed the pulmonary circulation.

It is also interesting to note that for thousands of years before its discovery in Europe the ancient Chinese believed in the circulation of blood. They were brought to this conclusion not by careful anatomical studies but for philosophical reasons. The *Nei Chin*, the classic Chinese medical text written around 2000 B.C., says that there are circular movements of both blood and energy in the body. The movement of the blood is controlled by the heart, that of the energy is controlled by the lungs. However, little advancement was made on these concepts as there was no tradition of surgery or human dissection in China. In addition, the limited contact between China and Europe would indicate the Chinese view probably had no influence on developments in the West.

In European medical schools the Vesalian tradition of the professor personally conducting the dissection was spreading. As more anatomists

---

19 Helen Rapson, *The Circulation of Blood, A History*. Frederick Muller Limited, London, 1982.

compared the words of Galen to their actual observations, more mistakes were uncovered. However, the concept of blood circulation was still not understood. Although a few advanced thinkers had discovered pulmonary circulation, their claims were not part of the mainstream. Ibn al-Nofis was unknown. All but three copies of Servetus' book were burned in 1553. It was essentially a 1559 textbook of Realdo Colombo, a student of Vesalius, that first demonstrated with experimental proof that the blood circulated from the right ventricle of the heart to the lungs and back to the left atrium. His widely read *De re anatomica* clearly established pulmonary circulation and published it to the world. He also noted there are four great vessels attached to the heart: two carry blood to the heart and two carry it away. Colombo also demonstrated that the valves in the heart keep the blood flowing in one direction. His book came very close to a complete description of the circulation of the blood, but he did not quite grasp that last concept.

The first clear statement of the circulation of blood published in European literature came from the Italian anatomist Cesalpino. He had studied medicine at Padua under Vesalius and became professor of anatomy at the University of Pisa. In 1593 Cesalpino published his book *Medical Questions* with experimental proof of the total circulation of blood. He demonstrated that blood flows from the heart through the arteries and back in the veins. He stated that there are "hair-like" vessels, which he called capillaries, that carry blood from the arteries to the veins.

Cesalpino demonstrated the existence of these vessels, which are invisible to the naked eye, by the following experiment: He exposed a vein of a living animal and tied it to stop the flow of blood. He then made a cut in the vein on the side of the ligature opposite the heart. The first blood to flow from the vein was dark (i.e., venous) blood, but soon brighter, arterial blood could be seen. The blood had to be coming from an artery feeding the vein.

Although he was the first to publish an accurate description of the circulation of blood, Cesalpino is seldom given credit for his pioneering work. He had the misfortune to be judged on his theological beliefs rather than his medical advances. His philosophical writings made him unacceptable to both Catholics and Protestants. His work was ignored, and credit for establishing the circulation of the blood and revolutionizing medicine went to an Englishman.

It was the very meticulous work of William Harvey that finally established the idea of continuous blood circulation in the body. Harvey, who had studied medicine at Cambridge, came to Padua in 1600 for two years for advanced study. From his teacher, Fabricus of Aquapendente, he learned that veins contain tiny valves that allow the blood to flow in one direction. Harvey returned to London where he practiced medicine until his death in 1657. In 1628 he published his short but monumental book *Exercitatio anatomica de motu cordis et sanguinis in animalibus* (An anatomical dissertation on the movement of the heart and blood in animals). His description of detailed experimental proofs established the basic concept of blood circulation that we believe in today. Since Harvey had studied in Italy, there is little doubt that he had heard of the work of Colombo and Cesalpino. However, he appears to have confirmed with his own experiments what he had heard, and he added further support to the concept with his own original calculations on the quantity of blood flowing in the body. By measuring the amount of blood expelled from the heart with each beat and multiplying that by the rate at which the heart beats, Harvey demonstrated that in one hour the heart pumps a quantity of blood equal to three times a person's weight. The volume of blood pumped by the heart is so great that it simply has to be recirculated in the body. For some reason he either did not hear of, or did not believe, the concept of capillaries connecting arteries and veins. He assumed that the blood passed from the arteries to the veins through some "porosities" in the flesh. It was necessary for the world to await the invention of the microscope before capillaries could be seen.

The Italian microscopist Marcello Malpighi (1628-1694) believed in Harvey's concept of the circulation of the blood and he looked for the connections between veins and arteries. He found the capillaries by looking at the very thin membranous material of a frog's lungs and reported his observations in 1661. That same year Anton van Leeuwenhoek used the microscope to make the first recorded observations of red cells.

In the eighteenth century, Anton Lavoisier, a French chemist, demonstrated that the respiration of living beings is a form of combustion – the reaction of oxygen with other materials. By the end of the century it had become apparent that as blood passes through the lungs oxygen is picked up and carbon dioxide is given off. However, there was still some doubt as to whether oxidation occurs in the lungs themselves or in some other part of the body. This question was finally settled in 1837 when Heinrich Gustav Magnus, a German chemist, demonstrated with his experiments that arterial blood contains more oxygen than venous blood and that the carbon dioxide in the venous blood has to come from the body tissues and is not created in the lungs.

The discovery that the blood circulates in the body and transports oxygen still left two questions unanswered: 1) What part or element in the blood is the main factor in this activity? and 2) Exactly how is the oxygen carried? Could the gases simply be dissolved in the liquid blood, or is there some component of the blood that binds to the oxygen and carries it to the cells?

The idea that oxygen might simply be dissolved in the blood is not an unreasonable one. When the surface of any liquid has a gas above it, the molecules of that gas will strike against the top of the liquid, and a certain number of gas molecules will dissolve in the liquid. However, liquids can hold only so many molecules of each gas, and soon molecules of gas will start to leave the liquid and return to the atmosphere above. An equilibrium point will be reached when the rate at which molecules are leaving the liquid equals the rate at which they are dissolving.

Not all gases have the same solubility in a liquid. Water exposed to the atmosphere will hold twice as much oxygen and 60 times as much carbon dioxide as nitrogen. (This high solubility of carbon dioxide makes possible the production of carbonated beverages.) In 1804 William Henry noted that for each particular gas the amount dissolved in a specific liquid depends strictly on the pressure of that gas above the liquid. The total pressure of all the gases above the liquid does not alter the solubility of the gas of interest. For example, the normal pressure of all gases in the atmosphere is expressed as 760 mm Hg. This is how high the atmosphere can push a column of mercury (Hg) in a barometer. This total pressure is the sum of the pressures exerted by all the gases in the atmosphere. Oxygen itself is responsible for about 160 mm Hg pressure. At this pressure a specific amount of oxygen will dissolve in water. If the oxygen pressure were to decrease to 80 mm Hg, half as much of the gas would dissolve in the water. Whether or not the total atmospheric pressure changes makes no difference. If the oxygen exerts 80 mm Hg pressure on the surface of the water, a specific amount of oxygen will dissolve in the water. It makes no difference if the rest of the gases combined add 100 or 700 mm Hg pressure.

A similar relationship holds if the water with the oxygen dissolved in it is separated by a gas permeable membrane from another liquid. There is a *tension* created in each liquid as a result of the efforts of the oxygen to leave the liquid. How great that tension is in one liquid depends on the amount of oxygen dissolved in it. Whether or not oxygen leaves one liquid and goes into the next depends on the solubility of oxygen in the two liquids and the actual amount of oxygen in each liquid. It does not depend on the other gases that may be dissolved in the liquids.

This approach to explaining gas transport would indicate that when the blood is exposed to air in the lungs, the pressure due to oxygen forces some $O_2$ molecules to dissolve in the blood. When the blood reaches the capillaries, where there is little, if any, $O_2$ tension, the oxygen leaves the blood and enters the cells. The blood would then return to the lungs with little or no oxygen, and the oxygen pressure in the lungs would cause more oxygen to dissolve in the blood.

The reverse would occur for carbon dioxide. As the waste gas is produced in the cells its tension would increase. When blood passes near the cells, the carbon dioxide would flow into the circulatory system. In the lungs the tension from $CO_2$ dissolved in the blood, which would be greater than the $CO_2$ pressure in the lungs, would push the gas out.

Experiments indicated that each liter of blood exposed to oxygen at the pressures found in the lungs should hold 3 mLs of oxygen. In fact, a liter of blood can actually contain up to 138 mLs of oxygen. Clearly the blood can carry more oxygen than would be expected as the result of simple solubility. This implies that something in the blood must be holding on to the oxygen. Mere solubility considerations can account for only 2% of the oxygen carried by the blood.

In the 1840's there were reports of observations of some type of crystalline material formed by the red pigment in blood. The crystals were analyzed and found to be proteins. In 1853 Ludwig Teichman, while a student at the University of Göttingen, separated from these red crystals a reddish-brown, non-protein substance that he called hemin. Teichman's procedure for preparing hemin was the first, and for many years the only, test to confirm the presence of blood on clothes and other objects. It became a standard test in forensic medicine.

During the 1860s some order was given to these observations on the red pigment in blood by a German physician and chemist, Dr. Felix Hoppe-Seyler. He had been born in 1825 as Felix Hoppe, the tenth child of a minister. Both his mother and father died when he was young, and he was raised by his older sister and her husband, Dr. Seyler. After completing his schooling he practiced medicine for several years. However, he found he preferred research, and from 1854 until his death in 1895 he held various teaching and research positions in German universities. In 1864 he was formally adopted by his guardians, and he changed his name to Hoppe-Seyler[20].

It was while he was a professor of applied chemistry at the Faculty of Medicine in Tübingen that Hoppe-Seyler did most of his research on hemoglobin. First, in 1864 he gave the substance the name that has stayed with it[21]. The word *hemoglobin*, like the compound itself, easily separates into two parts. Heme, which comes from the Greek word for blood, is a dark-red, iron-containing, non-protein compound. The other half, the globin, is the colorless protein left behind when heme is removed.

In addition to giving hemoglobin its name, Hoppe-Seyler also conducted some important studies on the color of blood. He introduced the newly invented spectroscope into medicine by using it to look at hemoglobin. Absorption spectroscopy, an important tool in the modern analytical lab, is based on the principle that solutions are colored because they absorb certain specific wavelengths of light and reflect others. When a solution changes color, it does so because there has been a change in the wavelengths of light that it absorbs. Hoppe-Seyler demonstrated that if light is passed through a solution of oxygenated hemoglobin, certain specific wavelengths (viz, 560 and 540 nm) will be absorbed. The result is the absorption pattern with two peaks seen in Figure 8.

---

20 E. Baumann and A. Kossel, "Zur Erinnerung an Felix Hoppe-Seyler," *Z. physiol. Chem.* 21:i-lxii, 1895-96

21 Felix Hoppe. "Über die chemischen und optischen Eigenschaften des Blutforbstoffs," *Archiv für pathologische Anatomis und Physiologie*, 29 (1864): 233-235.

## Figure 8. The Spectra of Hemoglobin

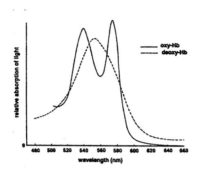

He found that oxygen loosely binds to hemoglobin to form oxyhemoglobin, which can give up its oxygen to the tissues in the body. He also confirmed the earlier observations of the French physiologist Claude Bernard that carbon monoxide is toxic because it displaces the oxygen from oxyhemoglobin.    Later, while a professor of physiological chemistry in Strasbourg, he demonstrated that chlorophyll, the green pigment in plants, has a structure similar to that of heme, the colored part of hemoglobin.  Felix Hoppe-Seyler's work laid such a strong foundation for further research on hemoglobin that it is not surprising that he is often referred to as the Father of Hemoglobin.

When G.G. Stokes, a British scientist, read Hoppe-Seyler's 1864 paper about hemoglobin and its absorption of certain wavelengths of light, it immediately occurred to him that he could use this property to study the changing color of blood in the body.  He found that as oxygen is removed from the blood, the two absorption peaks in the spectrum of the hemoglobin molecule disappear and are replaced by one single peak (i.e., the dotted line in Figure 8).  At the same time the color of the solution changes from red to purple.  If this purple solution is allowed to stand exposed to the air, it will change back to red and the two bands will return.   Thus, he correctly concluded, hemoglobin is capable of existing in two states — one containing more oxygen than the other.  When it passes from one state to the other, the color changes[22].

---

22 G. G. Stokes, "On the Reduction and Oxidation of the Colouring Matter of the Blood," *Proc. Roy. Soc. Lond.*, 13:355-364, 1864.

**Figure 9. The Hüfner and Bohr Curves**

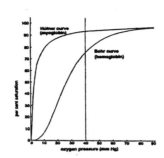

Stokes' experiments implied that the oxygen is not just dissolved in the blood. It actually reacts in some way with hemoglobin. This reaction occurs in the lungs and is reversed in the tissues of the body. This combination of oxygen and hemoglobin obviously had to be formed by a very loose bond so that the cycle could be repeated over and over. By the end of the nineteenth century the British biologist John Scott Haldane had demonstrated that carbon dioxide can undergo the same type of reaction with hemoglobin that oxygen does.

In 1890 Gustav Hüfner published an equation that predicted the behavior of hemoglobin under different oxygen pressures[23]. His equation was based strictly on calculations made from his experimental data. He found that if hemoglobin is exposed to a high concentration of oxygen, as it is in the lungs, it readily becomes saturated with oxygen. This means that the blood will quickly accept almost all the oxygen it can hold. However, in the capillaries there is little oxygen pressure and the hemoglobin molecules readily give up oxygen.

The relationship predicted by Hüfner is actually seen with myoglobin — a molecule one-fourth the size of hemoglobin that stores oxygen inside cells. However, some very careful studies published by Karl Hasselbach, August Krogh and Christian Bohr demonstrated that the behavior of hemoglobin actually differs slightly from that predicted by the Hüfner curve. The relationship between oxygen pressure and degree of saturation described by

---

23 G. Hüfner, "Ueber das Gesetz der Dissociation des Oxyhämoglobins und über einige daran sichknüpfenden wichtigen Fragen aus der Biologie," *Arch. Anat. Physiol. (Physiol. Abtheilung)* (1890), 1-27.

Hüfner results in a parabolic curve. The behavior of hemoglobin as determined by Bohr is a sigmoid (or S-shaped) curve. Both curves are depicted in Figure 9. The differences between the two curves are extremely important. In both theories the blood leaves the lungs, where the oxygen pressure is about 100 mm, completely saturated with oxygen. But, the amount of oxygen given up in the capillaries, where the typical oxygen pressure is 38 mm, is actually four times that predicted by the Hüfner curve. At 38 mm pressure the myoglobin will be about 92% saturated. This means it only yields about 8% of its oxygen. In contrast, hemoglobin will be 73% saturated – it will give up 27% of its oxygen at the pressure seen in the capillaries. The Bohr studies indicated that the hemoglobin molecule does a better job delivering oxygen to the cells than myoglobin would. While they both pick up the maximum amount of oxygen in the lungs, the hemoglobin will deliver more to the cells at the oxygen pressure that actually exists in the capillaries.

It was assumed that since the absorption of oxygen by the blood did not obey Henry's Law, as it would if the solubility of the gas in the liquid were the only factor, there must be some type of chemical bond formed between hemoglobin and oxygen. The nature of this bond and ease with which it seemed to be formed and broken did not fit the current concepts of chemical bonds. The most likely candidate for forming a bond with oxygen is the iron atom in the hemoglobin molecule. It was known to react readily with oxygen and was known to exist in two different oxidation states. Oxidation is a general term for a chemical reaction in which a substance loses an electron. If three electrons are removed from iron, it is said to be in the ferric ($Fe^{+3}$) state, e.g., as in the formation of ferric oxide (rust). A lower oxidation state, the ferrous ($Fe^{+2}$), occurs when only two electrons have been removed. Perhaps the iron in hemoglobin starts in the +2 state, reacts with oxygen and, in the process, loses an electron. Then it changes from +3 back to +2 when it gives up oxygen to the cells. Yet, the change between these two oxidation states was known even then to involve a great deal of energy, and the reaction is not easily reversed. There did not seem to be any reason why this reaction should proceed with such ease in the blood.

In 1923 a young U.S. chemist, James Bryant Conant, who later became President of Harvard, demonstrated experimentally that when oxygen combines with hemoglobin the iron atom starts out and remains in the ferrous

(+2) state[24]. This implies that during the uptake and release of oxygen the iron does not change oxidation states. The reaction is not a simple oxidation.

While Conant's work answered some of the questions, it still left unresolved the method by which hemoglobin can so readily pick up and release oxygen. If the iron atom does not change oxidation states, what part of the hemoglobin actually holds on to the oxygen molecule? Understanding this process had to await the complete details of the structure of the hemoglobin molecule.

---

24 J. B. Conant, "An Electrochemical Study of Hemoglobin," *J. Biol. Chem.* 57:401-414, 1923.

*Chapter 3*

# THE SEARCH FOR STRUCTURE

As more details were discovered about the function of hemoglobin in the body, additional questions naturally arose concerning its structure. Teichman had demonstrated that the molecule separated into two different substances: the red, iron-containing heme and the clear globin, a protein. This opened the question as to how the two substances actually combine and work together to give hemoglobin its unusual properties.

Exactly how many atoms does each molecule of hemoglobin have? What atoms are they, how are they arranged, and why does this arrangement give hemoglobin its unusual ability to pick up oxygen without actually oxidizing the iron? And what are the exact size and shape of the hemoglobin molecule?

The first problem to be solved was to determine exactly how many and what kinds of atoms make up one hemoglobin molecule. The earliest careful elemental analysis of the chemical composition of hemoglobin was reported in 1885 by O. Zinoffsky in Basil, Switzerland. His study of horse hemoglobin indicated that for each iron atom there are 712 carbon (C), 1,130 hydrogen (H), 214 nitrogen (N), 245 oxygen (O) and 2 sulfur (S) atoms. This means that hemoglobin has the basic formula $C_{712}H_{1130}N_{214}O_{245}S_2Fe$ with a molecular weight of 16,730[†].

However, this basic formula and weight assume that hemoglobin contains only one iron atom. If, in fact, it contains more than one, then the actual molecular weight will be a multiple of 16,730.

---

† The correct unit for molecular weight is "daltons," but it is usually omitted.

Two men in two different countries using two entirely different methods came independently to the same conclusion that there are four iron atoms in one molecule of human hemoglobin and its molecular weight is about 67,000.

G.S. Adair in Cambridge used osmotic pressure measurements to determine the molecular weight of hemoglobin. To perform these measurements Adair placed a solution of hemoglobin in a bag made from a material called collodion membrane. (Figure 10.) This membrane contains pores that are small enough for water and salts to pass through but not big enough to permit passage of the larger hemoglobin molecules. The bag is first filled with a solution of hemoglobin. The top of the bag is wrapped around and sealed to a long glass tube. It is then placed in a jar of water with the tube sticking into the air above the water. The water in the jar pushes into the bag in an effort to dilute the hemoglobin solution. The driving force for this is called osmotic pressure. Water will keep forcing itself into the bag until the bag swells out and pressure from the membrane starts pushing water out of the collodion bag and back into the jar.

## Figure 10. Measurement of Osmotic Pressure

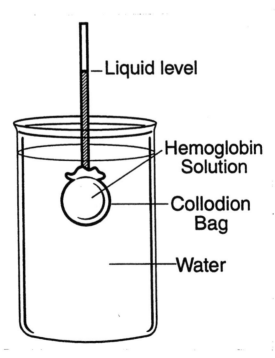

Soon the pressure of the membrane pushing water out is equal to the osmotic pressure forcing it in. When this equilibrium is reached, the pressure in the bag is indicated by the height to which the water has risen in the tube. The system is somewhat analogous to the measurement of temperature with a thermometer. In this case, however, the height of the column of liquid is related to the pressure inside the bag. Because the pressure changes with the size of the molecule dissolved in the water in the bag, the height of the liquid can be used to estimate the molecular weight of the material in the solution enclosed in the collodion membrane. Adair carried out these osmotic pressure studies on hemoglobin and reported in 1925 that it has a molecular weight of 67,000.

During roughly the same period a Swedish chemist, Theodore Svedberg, developed a new instrument called the ultracentrifuge. In a typical laboratory centrifuge, tubes filled with solutions are spun in a circle at speeds that create forces equivalent to between a few hundred and a few thousand times the force of gravity. The ultracentrifuge creates forces up to 20,000 times the force of gravity. The normal centrifuge can be used to precipitate large particles from a solution, e.g., it will pack down at the bottom of the tube the red and white cells in blood. The ultracentrifuge running at high speeds for several days can actually separate large molecules that have been dissolved in the right solution. Svedberg found that if he placed proteins in a tube with a dense sucrose solution and spun it in a circle at very high speeds, he could estimate the molecular weight of the protein by measuring its position after several days in the ultracentrifuge. The first protein Svedberg studied was hemoglobin, and he found it had a molecular weight of approximately 68,000. This implied four iron-containing units. His results were published in 1926.

To determine the exact arrangement of the atoms in hemoglobin took many scientists working over a period of about 30 years. There were essentially three problems to be solved. While research into all three was going on at the same time during the 1930s, 1940s and 1950s, each problem was essentially approached and solved separately. First, it was necessary to determine the structure of heme, the iron containing portion of the hemoglobin. Then it was necessary to find the composition of the protein chain. Since proteins are made of amino acids combined in a long chain, this meant finding the exact sequences of amino acids that formed globin. Finally, the three-dimensional fit of the two separate units, the heme and the globin, had to be determined by x-ray analysis.

## Figure 11. Pyrolle

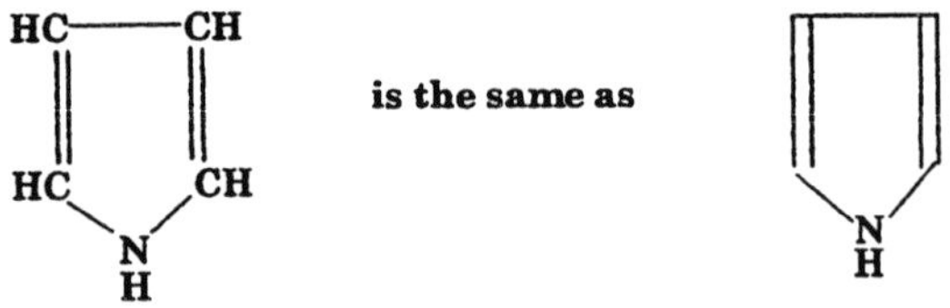

Heme was found to belong to a class of compounds called iron porphyrins. Its structure was determined by W. Kuster in 1912 and reported in the biochemical research journal established by Hoppe-Seyler.[25] The chemistry and synthesis of heme, as well as that of many other metal porphyrins, was investigated in greater detail by Hans Fischer and his associates in Munich between 1920 and 1940. Porphyrin compounds include two of the most important molecules in nature: hemoglobin and chlorophyll. The first is responsible for respiration in animals; the second is required for photosynthesis in plants. The basic unit of the porphyrin system of compounds is the pyrolle ring. This ring contains four carbon and one nitrogen atom arranged in a circle. There is a hydrogen attached to each of the ring atoms, and two pairs of carbons are joined with a double bond (-C=C-). (See Figure 11.) To simplify the notation, the structure is often written without actually indicating the carbon atoms or any hydrogen atoms that are attached to carbon atoms. They are assumed to be there. However, the presence of any double bonds, any nitrogen atoms, and hydrogens attached to nitrogens is always noted. The basic representation of the pyrolle ring is also illustrated in Figure 11.

In the formation of a porphyrin, four of these pyrolle rings are joined into a circle with the nitrogens in the center. Each pyrolle is linked to the next by means of a carbon bridge ( =C- ). In two of the pyrolle rings the hydrogen has been removed from the nitrogen and there is the formation and rearrangement of double bonds. The net result, using the simplified notation, is given in Figure 12.

---

25 W. Kunster, "Beitrage zur Kenntnis des Bilirubins und Hömins," *Hoppe-Seyler's Z. Physiol. Chem.* 82:463, 1912.

## Figure 12. Porphyrin

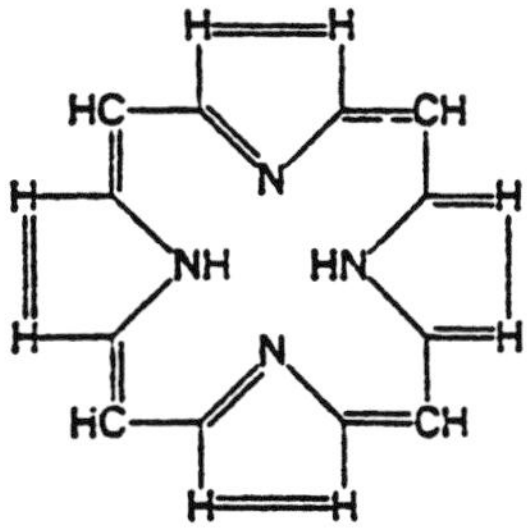

Metalloporphyrins have a metal atom (e.g., copper, iron or magnesium) in the center with bonds to the four nitrogens. There are also different side groups attached to various pyrolle rings — exactly which groups depends on the particular compound. The structure of heme and chlorophyll are in Figure 13. Notice the striking similarity in the structures of these two molecules. Each heme molecule contains a ring of four porphyrins with an iron (Fe) in the middle; each chlorophyll contains a ring of four porphyrins with a magnesium (Mg) in the middle.

The unraveling of the globin chain structure was accomplished next. Proteins all have the same basic structure: they are long chains of various amino acids linked together. The challenge is to determine the exact sequence of amino acids that goes into the formation of a particular protein.

## Figure 13. Heme and Chlorophyll

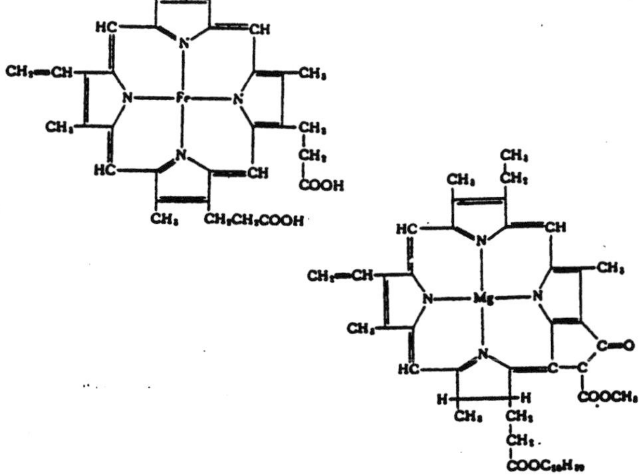

**Figure 14. An Amino Acid**

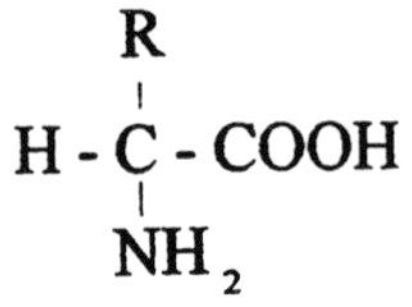

$$R$$
$$H - C - COOH$$
$$NH_2$$

All amino acids have a carbon atom with two groups attached. One group, called the carboxylic acid, consists of another carbon with two oxygens and a hydrogen. By itself the carboxylic acid is written -COOH. The second group, the amine, is a nitrogen with two hydrogens. Its symbol is $-NH_2$. The general structure for an amino acid in shown in Figure 14. The -R indicates a different group that changes for each specific amino acid. For example, when -R is a hydrogen atom by itself, the amino acid is glycine. When -R is the methyl group ($-CH_3$), the amino acid is alanine. A list of the most common amino acids will be found in Table I.

Amino acids have the property of being able to join together to form long chains, called peptides, and even longer chains, called proteins. A typical protein will contain hundreds of amino acids arranged in a long chain in a specific sequence. The exact sequence of the amino acids is critical. In a protein with 150 amino acids, the replacement of one amino acid for another can significantly alter the properties of the molecule. It can, in the human body, make a difference between sickness and health, between life and death.

Because the exact sequence of amino acids is so critical, a simple elemental analysis of a protein provides little useful information. It is not enough to know how many carbon, hydrogen, oxygen, nitrogen, and sulfur atoms are in the protein. It is necessary to determine the exact sequence of amino acids in the protein to distinguish one from another. The globin part of hemoglobin was found to contain four separate chains of amino acids. Two of the chains were identical, and each one contained 141 amino acids. The other two were also identical to each other but had 146 amino acids. The first was designated the alpha chain; the second was called the beta chain.

## Table I: The Amino Acids in Hemoglobin

| Amino Acid | Abbreviation |
|---|---|
| Alanine | Ala |
| Arginine | Arg |
| Asparagine | Asn |
| Aspartic Acid | Asp |
| Cysteine | Cys |
| Glutamic Acid | Glu |
| Glutamine | Gln |
| Glycine | Gly |
| Histidine | His |
| Isoleucine | Ile |
| Leucine | Leu |
| Lysine | Lys |
| Methionine | Met |
| Phenylalanine | Phe |
| Proline | Pro |
| Serine | Ser |
| Threonine | Thr |
| Tryptophane | Trp |
| Tyrosine | Tyr |
| Valine | Val |

**Figure 15. Amino Acid Sequence of Alpha Chains**

*A→*
val-leu-ser-pro-ala-asp-lys-thr-asn-val-lys-ala-ala-try-gly-

*B→*
lys-val-gly-ala-his-ala-gly-glu-tyr-gly-ala-glu-ala-leu-glu-

*C→*
arg-met-phe-leu-ser-phe-pro-thr-thr-lys-thr-phe-pro-his-

*D→*               *E→*
phe-asp-leu-ser-his-gly-ser-ala-gln-val-lys-gly-his-gly-

lys-lys-val-ala-asp-ala-leu-thr-asn-ala-val-ala-

*F→*
his-val-asp-asp-met-pro-asn-ala-leu-ser-ala-leu-ser-asp-

*G→*
leu-his-ala-his-lys-leu-arg-val-asp-pro-val-asn-phe-lys-

leu-leu-ser-his-cys-leu-leu-val-thr-leu-ala-ala-his-

*H→*
leu-pro-ala-glu-phe-thr-pro-ala-val-his-ala-ser-leu-asp-

lys-phe-phe-ala-ser-val-ser-thr-val-leu-thr-ser-

lys-tyr-arg

**Figure 16. The Amino Acid Sequence of Beta Chains**

*A*→
val-his-leu-thr-pro-glu-glu-lys-ser-ala-val-thr-ala-leu-try-

*B*→
gly-lys-val-asn-val-asp-glu-val-gly-gly-glu-ala-leu-gly-

*C*→
arg-leu-leu-val-val-tyr-pro-try-thr-gln-arg-phe-pro-thr-

*D*→                    *E*→
phe-glu-ser-phe-gly-asp-leu-ser-thr-pro-asp-ala-val-met-

gly-asn-pro-lys-val-lys-ala-his-gly-lys-lys-

val-leu-gly-ala-phe-ser-asp-gly-leu-ala-his-leu-asp-asn-

*F*→
leu-lys-gly-thr-phe-ala-thr-leu-ser-glu-leu-his-cys-asp-lys-

*G*→
leu-his-val-asp-pro-glu-asn-phe-arg-leu-leu-gly-asn-val-

*H*→
leu-val-cys-val-leu-ala-his-his-phe-gly-lys-glu-phe-thr-

pro-pro-val-gln-ala-ala-tyr-gln-lys-val-val-ala-gly-val-ala-

asn-ala-asn-ala-leu-ala-his-lys-tyr-his

The exact amino acid sequences of the two chains were determined by the efforts of several groups of investigators: Gerhardt Braunitzer and his colleagues at the Max Plank Institute for Biochemistry in Munich; William Konigsberg, Robert Hill and their associates at the Rockefeller Institute in New York; Rhinesmith, Schroeder, and Pauling in California; Ingram in England. The amino acid sequence of the alpha ($\alpha$) chain is given in Figure 15 and that of the beta ($\beta$) chain in Figure 16. The alphabetical sections (A, B, C, etc.) indicated in the diagram are arbitrary divisions to place the amino acids in the various sections of the protein as it twists and turns to create a pocket for the heme. These sections are illustrated in the three-dimensional representation of a globin chain seen in Figure 17. Sections A and H are long, straight segments of the chain, B, C, and D are short curved segments, and F is the section of the chain nearest the heme.

**Figure 17. One Heme-globin Unit**

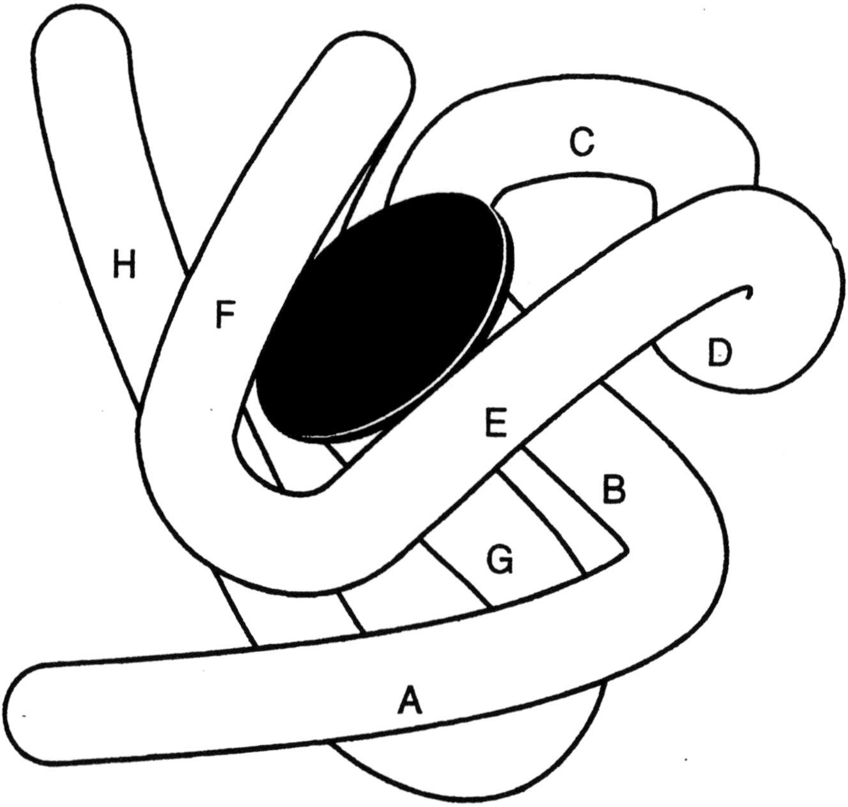

The third approach to the analysis of the structure of hemoglobin involved determining the actual three dimensional arrangement of atoms. It was basically the responsibility of one man: Max Perutz. In 1937 Max Perutz entered Cambridge University as a graduate student from Austria. Only the year before J. D. Bernal, working in the Cavandish Laboratory at Cambridge, had discovered that proteins could be made to crystallize and their structure studied using x-ray analysis. There was a great deal of excitement about this at the time and many scientists began to explore the potential applications of this discovery. John Kendrew and his collaborators at Cambridge were looking into the structure of myoglobin (the molecule that transports oxygen around the inside of cells). When Perutz joined Kendrew's group, he selected the x-ray analysis of hemoglobin for his research project. Not only did he realize the physiological importance of hemoglobin, but he knew that it had already been established that hemoglobin could be crystallized.

**Figure 18. The Hemoglobin Molecule**

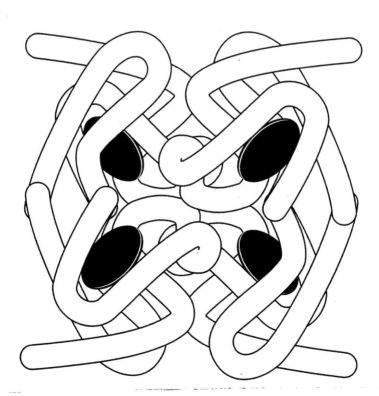

Although he did receive his doctorate for his research after a few years, it actually took about 23 years for Perutz and his coworkers to determine the very complicated three dimensional structure of hemoglobin. In x-ray analysis the crystals of a protein are mounted wet in a small glass capillary tube. A narrow beam of x-rays is then focused on the crystals. The x-rays strike the crystals and are deflected in a specific pattern that can be mathematically related to the arrangement of atoms in the hemoglobin molecule. During the investigations into the structure of hemoglobin it was necessary to analyze several thousand x-ray diffraction patterns. The picture that eventually emerged indicated that each heme unit is surrounded by one of the globin chains. The globin coils around in such a manner as to form a small pocket in which a flat, disc-shaped heme sits. (Figure 17.) The four heme-globin units then combine to make one hemoglobin molecule with four heme groups nestled into separate pockets: two in alpha chains and two in beta chains. (See Figure 18.) While the alpha and beta chains are not actually connected to each other, there are some very important weak bonds, called salt bridges, holding them together. These salt bridges are weak electrostatic bonds formed when there is a negative charge on an amino acid in one globin chain. This negative charge is weakly attracted to an amino acid on the opposite globin if their arrangement brings them close together. The attraction between the two amino acids is not strong enough to form a covalent band, the type of strong chemical bond that holds together atoms in a typical molecule like the carbon-carbon bond in an amino acid, but it is strong enough to create some resistance to moving the two amino acids away from each other. (Figure 19.)

When the hemoglobin molecule is without oxygen (i.e., it is deoxyhemoglobin) it is in a tighter, more compact configuration known as the tense, or T, state. In this position an aspartic acid on the beta chain finds itself opposite a tyrosine molecule on the alpha chain. The aspartic acid has a negative charge because there is a tendency for the -COOH group to ionize, giving off $H^+$ ions and leaving -COO$^-$. This negative charge exerts a pull on a hydrogen atom that is part of a tyrosine on the alpha chain. While the aspartic acid cannot pull the H completely away from the tyrosine, it does hold on to it with a weak bond.

## Figure 19. Salt Bridges Between Globin Chains

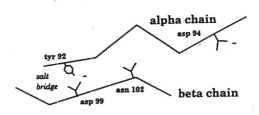

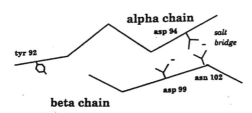

After it has picked up oxygen the hemoglobin molecule shifts to a slightly looser, or relaxed, configuration known as the R state. The globins move slightly, and in this position the aspartic acid is no longer across from the tyrosine. The salt bridge has been broken. However, now an aspartic acid on the alpha chain find itself across from an asparagine on the beta chain. Once again a salt bridge is formed that holds the two chains together. Thus the molecule can slip from one position to the next, back and forth, as salt bridges are broken and formed.

But, why should the chains move from one state to the next? There must be some force that breaks the bond at one position and moves the chains to permit formation of salt bridges at a new location. How can the attachment of oxygen to the hemoglobin alter these salt bridges? While the iron is located in the flat, planar structure of the heme and is surrounded by porphyrin rings to which it is bound, it also forms a bond with one particular amino acid on the globin chain. Each globin chain has a histidine molecule (called the 'proximal' histidine) located directly under the iron atom. The histidine has a ring of atoms with nitrogen in it, similar to the porphyrin rings, and one of these nitrogens forms a bond with the iron atom. When there is no oxygen on the hemoglobin molecule, the proximal histidine pulls the iron into the hemoglobin. This iron is, of course, still bound to the porphyrin rings in the heme, so this attraction bends the heme plane very slightly. When oxygen is bonded to the iron, it "pops" the iron back into the flat heme plane. (Figure 20.) This motion pulls this histidine with it. The movement of the histidine is transmitted along the globin chain. This breaks the T-state salt bridges and permits formation of R-state salt bridges.

The presence or absence of oxygen influences the position of iron with respect to porphyrin rings in the heme. This, in turn, alters the position of the proximal histidine, the configuration of the globin chains, and the types of salt bridges formed. In a like manner, anything that causes a change in the salt bridge will either pull the iron into the hemoglobin molecule, causing it to give up oxygen, or push it out, making it available for attachment to oxygen. Thus the gain or loss of oxygen from one point on the hemoglobin alters the entire structure of the molecule and encourages rapid transformation back and forth between the conditions of oxygenation and deoxygenation. Perutz likened this change to the action of a miniature lung. He called hemoglobin a "breathing molecule" that, contrary to what we might anticipate, expands when it gives off oxygen and contracts when oxygen is taken up[26].

### Figure 20. Movement of the Heme Plane

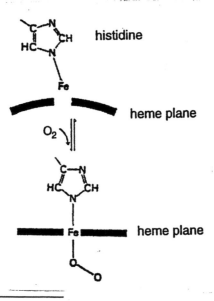

---

26 M. F. Perutz, "The hemoglobin molecule," *Scientific American* 234: 64-76, Nov 1964.

When there is an abundance of oxygen, as in the lungs, the gas molecules attach themselves to the iron. In the capillaries in the tissues of the body, where there is less oxygen, the gas is given up. A single heme-globin unit, like myoglobin, would do this, but four such units acting in concert can do a better job. As oxygen molecules join and leave an iron, the metal atom moves in and out of the heme plane. This movement changes the extent of the pull the iron has on the histidine. Movement of the histidine translates along the protein chain to make and break salt bridges. This, in turn, forces neighboring iron atoms to move in an out of their heme planes. Irons pushed out of the plane are exposed and ready to pick up oxygen. Iron atoms pulled into the plane quickly release oxygen.

This heme-heme interaction explains the Bohr effect and is responsible for hemoglobin's ability to so readily pick up oxygen in the lungs and then so readily give it up to the cells. A single heme-globin unit could be used for oxygen transport in the blood, but four acting together as a hemoglobin molecule can carry more oxygen to the cells with greater efficiency.

# Chapter 4

# HEMOGLOBIN AT WORK

The picture that has emerged from the last one hundred years of research on the structure and function of hemoglobin is that of a highly specialized molecule that is specifically designed to serve the greatest need of the human body — an immediate, ample supply of oxygen to every cell. The human body has at its disposal a very complex mechanism to assure that hemoglobin is available in the quantities and places needed. It does not look to an outside nutritional source for this substance but manufactures it itself to its own specifications. The only job it must perform is to aid in the transport of gases (oxygen and carbon dioxide).

This need for a constant supply of oxygen is not limited to humans. It is essential for every animal from the single-cell protozoa, fish and insects to mice, humans and elephants. Animals need oxygen to live. It is the reaction of oxygen with carbon compounds that provides the energy necessary to maintain life.

These reactions between oxygen and carbon compounds, like sugars, take place in cellular components called mitochondria. There food is oxidized, and the energy released in the process is stored in other molecules that the cell can use when needed. At the same time, carbon dioxide ($CO_2$) is created as a waste by-product of the chemical reactions that release the energy. This creates a new problem as $CO_2$ can inhibit cellular activity and must be removed from the cell as soon as possible. Organisms have two gas transport problems – bringing oxygen to the cells and taking away carbon dioxide.

For oxygen to reach the single-cell organism it must first leave the air and dissolve in water. Then it must diffuse through the water until it reaches the membrane surrounding the cell. Finally, it must pass through the cell's outer membrane into the liquid cytoplasm where it is stored until needed by the mitochondria. As organisms become larger and more complex this process is inadequate. Larger animals quickly use up the oxygen in their vicinity and need a greater supply than can be provided by simple diffusion through the watery environment in which they live. The organism must either bring in new sources of oxygen or move itself to a region with a new supply of oxygen.

For example, fish have gills to remove oxygen from the water in which they live. Most fish bring water in through their mouths then close them and use their muscles to force the water across the gills. The gills extract oxygen and dump carbon dioxide before the water is expelled from the body. Other fish, like the mackerel and the tuna, swim with their mouths open and use the force generated by their forward motion to push the water past the gills. If they did not constantly move forward they would soon die of asphyxiation.

During the Devonian Period (some 400 million years ago) amphibians began to leave the sea, move onto the land, and use air itself as a source for oxygen. It may have been that the warm, swampy waters were low in oxygen and some fish needed to rise to the surface to catch small bubbles of air. Soon animals with lungs evolved. The air contains 20 times more oxygen than water, and the gas can diffuse through it one million times faster than through water. Air can provide a richer, more readily accessible supply of oxygen than can water. A wide variety of large, land based animals eventually evolved.

Once acquired by the animal, however, the oxygen must still be distributed to each cell in the body. Meanwhile the problem of removal of the poisonous $CO_2$ has become more difficult. As animals increased in size and moved onto the land, the solution to these problems became more complex. There are still some multi-celled organisms that rely on diffusion through water to supply oxygen to all their individual cells and that let the wastes be removed by diffusion away from the cells. The jellyfish, for example, can do this because it has a low rate of activity (hence, no need for a ready supply of large amounts of oxygen) and a high (~99%) water content. Other animals, like insects, rely on diffusion but employ a complex system of hollow tubes to bring air directly to the cells. Most animals, however, developed a system to circulate a liquid that contains the oxygen and then carries off the carbon dioxide. The oxygen is not simply dissolved in the liquid. It is, instead, attached to special molecules that transport it through the body and can then be used to remove the carbon dioxide. Because these molecules that transport gases are usually colored, they are referred to collectively as respiratory pigments.

We do not know how many respiratory pigments were developed and discarded during the course of the evolution of life on earth. However, hemoglobin seems to have developed early and is so well suited for the job that it has become the most widespread of the respiratory pigments. There are some copper-based respiratory pigments, those found in squid and octopus, for example, and two other iron-containing respiratory pigments found in a few invertebrates, but no other molecule has proven to satisfy the critical gas transport function as well as hemoglobin. It is found in trace amounts in some microorganisms, e.g., in the Paramecium and in some molds, but we don't know exactly how it functions and its purpose for being there. There is also a hemoglobin-like molecule that is an important component of the root nodules of legumes (e.g., peas and peanuts) where it seems to be involved in the process of nitrogen fixation.

In invertebrates the respiratory pigment floats freely in the circulating liquid. In vertebrates it is packed into cells that are swept along by the circulating liquid. The cells are alternately exposed to oxygen in the lungs (or gills) and then taken to the various tissues of the body where they give up oxygen and pick up carbon dioxide. The blood cells that contain respiratory pigments are amazingly similar in size and design for all vertebrates. (See Figure 21.)

### Figure 21. Red Blood Cells of Vertebrates

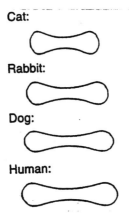

Cat:

Rabbit:

Dog:

Human:

## Figure 22. The Respiratory System

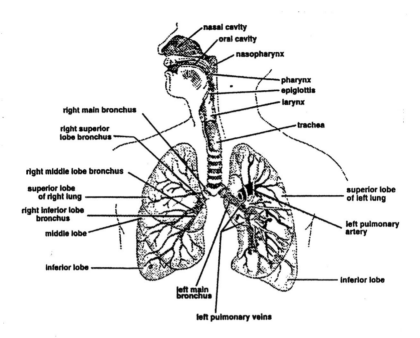

## Figure 23. The Alveolus

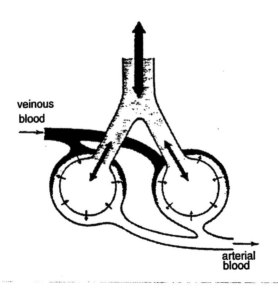

In humans the air enters the body through the nose and mouth and passes into the trachea. The trachea splits into the right and left bronchial tubes that take the air to the lungs. In the lungs the bronchial tubes split into branches, divide, and further subdivide into smaller and smaller vessels. At the end of this passageway the air is sucked into small chambers called alveoli. There are approximately 300 million alveoli in each lung, and it is here that gas exchange with the blood takes place. Each alveolus has a membrane wall that is only 0.3 mm thick. The transfer of oxygen from the lungs to the blood and of carbon dioxide from the blood to the lungs takes place across this membrane. Although each alveolus is very small, the total surface area of alveolar membrane in the average human adult is 50-100 square meters (approximately 500 – 1,000 square feet).

Each alveolar sack is surrounded by a capillary that brings venous blood from the heart (via the pulmonary artery). Although it flows through an artery, it is called venous blood because it is low in oxygen and high in carbon dioxide like the blood in veins. This blood enters the space around the membrane that surrounds the alveolus. Oxygen and carbon dioxide can diffuse through this membrane. The blood leaving the alveolar sack, called arterial because it is now rich in oxygen and low in carbon dioxide, is returned to the heart to be distributed to the rest of the body.

In a mixture of two or more gases, each gas will diffuse throughout the container and exert a pressure on the surrounding walls. The pressure exerted by each gas depends solely on its concentration and not on the concentration of the other gases. In following the changes in the amounts of oxygen and carbon dioxide in the lungs, blood, and tissues of the body, we need some way to express relative concentrations. The easiest way to do this is to talk about the pressure exerted by the gas at each stage of the process.

For example, the gases in the air are said to exert a total pressure of one atmosphere. We can measure air pressure by using a tube filled with mercury (Hg) as a barometer. If there is no air pushing down on the top of the mercury column (i.e., there is a vacuum in the tube) one atmosphere of air pressure can push a column of mercury to a height of 760 mm. Thus the pressure of all the gases in the air is said to equal 760 mm Hg. Since each gas exerts pressure independently, each adds to the total pressure in proportion to its concentration. Thus nitrogen, which accounts for 78% of the air, is responsible for

$$760 \times 0.78 = 593 \text{ mm Hg.}$$

That is, $pN_2 = 593$ mm Hg in air[†]. Likewise, in air $pO_2 = 760 \times 0.2071 = 157$ mm Hg and $pCO_2 = 0.3$ mm Hg.

In summary the air we breathe in has the following composition by pressure (mm of Hg).

$$pN_2 \ = \ 593$$
$$pO_2 \ = \ 157$$
$$pCO_2 \ = \ 0.3$$
$$pH_2O \ = \ 9.5$$

The air coming into the lungs mixes with that already there. It does not come in, exchange gases with the blood, then move out. There is constant intermixing. Hence, the gas composition tends to reach a steady state that reflects the sum of all that is happening.

If we measure the air in the alveolar sack, we find the following:

$$pN_2 \ = \ 574$$
$$pO_2 \ = \ 100$$
$$pCO_2 \ = \ 40$$
$$pH_2O \ = \ 45$$

As we would expect, the oxygen concentration has decreased. Fresh air brings in new oxygen, but it is continually being removed by the blood. On the other hand, the $CO_2$ concentration in the alveolar sack is very high. It is also a very moist environment, so the pressure due to water vapor is high.

The gas leaving the body has the following average composition:

$$pN_2 \ = \ 574$$
$$pO_2 \ = \ 111$$
$$pCO_2 \ = \ 30$$
$$pH_2O \ = \ 45$$

---

† The lower case "p" indicates the "partial pressure" due to that gas. Thus, pO2 is the partial pressure due to oxygen.

Not unexpectedly we can conclude that the air we breathe out has less oxygen and more carbon dioxide than the air we breathe in.

The blood coming into contact with the alveolar sack contains oxygen and carbon dioxide. The oxygen is present in two forms and the carbon dioxide in three. Most oxygen is, of course, attached to hemoglobin molecules in the red cell. However, a small percentage is simply dissolved in the blood plasma. Carbon dioxide is transported through the blood in three forms: as dissolved $CO_2$, as bicarbonate ion, or attached to hemoglobin.

The $CO_2$ dissolved in the plasma can freely pass through the membrane surrounding the red cell and diffuse into the cytoplasm, the liquid interior of the cell. Carbon dioxide dissolved in water will react with the $H_2O$ molecules and form carbonic acid ($H_2CO_3$). However, in the cytoplasm of the red cell is an enzyme, carbonic anhydrase, that speeds up this reaction and accelerates the rate at which it occurs by a factor of one million. After the carbonic acid has been formed, it readily disassociates into two ions, hydrogen ion ($H^+$) and bicarbonate ions ($HCO_3^-$). This bicarbonate is the same as that found in sodium bicarbonate, baking soda. Because the carbonic anhydrase promotes the rapid conversion of carbon dioxide to carbonic acid ($H_2CO_3$), the $CO_2$ is able to dissolve so readily in the blood. Approximately two-thirds of the $CO_2$ in venous blood is in the form of bicarbonate ion. Some bicarbonate will be formed in the plasma, but most is created in the red cell and diffuses out to the plasma. Finally, some of the dissolved $CO_2$ will actually react with free, uncharged amino groups on the hemoglobin molecule to form carbaminohemoglobin.

Venous blood approaching the alveolus has $pO_2 = 38$ and $pCO_2 = 46$. The higher pressure oxygen in the alveolus (100 mm Hg) pushes across the membrane to dissolve in the plasma. Oxygen in the plasma diffuses into the red cell and reacts with hemoglobin. When the first oxygen reacts with a deoxyhemoglobin molecule, it "pulls" an iron atom away from the histidine. This motion forces the breakage of salt bridges and the molecule returns to the R state. As more oxygen is picked up, more diffuses into the red cell from the plasma, leaving room for more oxygen to enter the plasma across the alveolar membrane. This continues until the $pO_2$ of the blood leaving the lung is equal to the $pO_2$ of the air in the sack (i.e., 100 mm Hg).

When the hemoglobin molecule passes from the T to the R state, hydrogen ions ($H^+$) are given off as the salt bridges break. These $H^+$ ions react with $HCO_3^-$ to form carbonic acid. The carbonic acid then decomposes to

$H_2O$ and $CO_2$. The blood approaching the alveolus has $pCO_2 = 46$, slightly higher than the $pCO_2$ of 40 mm Hg in the alveolus. Hence $CO_2$ will pass from the blood across the alveolar membrane to the alveolus. As $CO_2$ is formed from the decomposition of carbonic acid, it dissolves in the plasma and passes into the alveolus. This process continues until the $pCO_2$ of the blood equals the $pCO_2$ in the alveolus (i.e., 40 mm Hg).

Thus these processes reinforce each other. The increase in oxygen causes the transformation of hemoglobin from the T to the R state. Reaction of one oxygen with one hemoglobin breaks salt bridges and the molecules push out the iron atom to encourage reaction with more oxygens. Meanwhile, the broken salt bridges have released $H^+$ ions that react with bicarbonate to produce $CO_2$. This increases pressure from $CO_2$ and diffusion of $CO_2$ into the alveolus.

The red cells pass through the arteries and into the capillaries that are positioned next to body cells. Each hemoglobin molecule is holding onto four oxygen molecules, and there is a small amount of oxygen dissolved in the plasma. The body cells are very low in oxygen and the $pO_2$ is very low. Oxygen from the blood diffuses across the capillary membrane into the cells. Oxygen starts to leave hemoglobin to replace that lost from the plasma.

When the first oxygen leaves, the iron to which it was attached "pops" back into the heme. This movement is translated along the globin chain and encourages the formation of new salt bridges as the molecule goes from the R to the T state. To complete the formation of the salt bridges there is pressure on the other heme units to give up their oxygen. Once the first oxygen is lost there is a quick release of the other three.

There is low oxygen pressure in the cell because it has been captured by myoglobin for storage until needed in metabolic processes. When the oxygen is used, carbon dioxide is created. The increased $CO_2$ pressure in the cell forces $CO_2$ across the capillary membrane and into the blood. There it can diffuse into the red cell where it forms carbonic acid, which yields hydrogen ions ($H^+$) and bicarbonate ion ($HCO_3^-$).

The bicarbonate ion is readily soluble in water. Only by converting $CO_2$ to this form can the body remove large quantities of the waste gas from the cell. However, in the formation of the bicarbonate ions there are hydrogen ions created. These ions will make the blood dangerously acidic unless there is something there to absorb and neutralize excess $H^+$. Fortunately, when hemoglobin moves to its T state and new salt bridges are formed, sites are made available to bond with the hydrogen ions. These sites will still have a positive charge to offset the negative charge on the bicarbonate ion. This keeps the net charge neutral without, however, generating free $H^+$ ions in the blood.

Once the mechanism and the chemistry of the process of gas transport is understood, it is possible to appreciate the implications of the Hüfner and Bohr curves. Refer again to the two curves in Figure 9, Chapter 2.

The pressure of oxygen in the lungs stays at 100 mm while in the capillaries it is 40. Under normal conditions these two values don't change. They are the steady-state result of all the processes occurring simultaneously. In the alveolus $CO_2$ is brought in by the blood, oxygen is being carried off by the blood, and the gas mixture in the chamber is partially exhaled and then replenished with fresh air. If we were to monitor the pressure in the alveolus we would see that it does not change. The pressure of the gases and the concentration of each gas remains constant during the respiratory process. Oxygen pressure stays at 100; carbon dioxide at 40.

Likewise, in the capillaries the oxygen pressure stays at 40 mm. This is the sum of all the activities: gas entering the cell, leaving the cell, dissolving in the serum, and reacting with hemoglobin. The Hüfner curve and the Bohr curve reveal that at an oxygen pressure of 100 mm Hg both myoglobin and hemoglobin will be saturated. They will both pick up all the oxygen they can hold. At 40 mm, however, the two curves are quite different. If myoglobin (which is, essentially, one heme-globin unit) were to transport oxygen in the blood, it would give up about 8% of its load to the cells, if the pressure were 40. In other words, 92% of the myoglobin would return to the lungs with the oxygen still attached. Hemoglobin is about 73% saturated at 40 mm, so it gives up 27% of its oxygen and returns to the lungs with 73%.

While hemoglobin will release more oxygen in the capillaries, it is important to remember that three fourths of the hemoglobin molecules have oxygen attached to them while in the veins returning to the lungs. This creates a large reservoir of oxygen in the blood that the body can draw on if necessary. To see how this can occur, look again at the curves. Notice the behavior of myoglobin as the oxygen pressure decreases. If myoglobin were used to carry oxygen in the blood and the oxygen pressure in the capillaries dropped below 40, the myoglobin would undergo only a very small change in its degree of saturation. It would not readily give up more oxygen. Inside the cell, where the myoglobin does its work, if there is a serious drop in oxygen pressure and an immediate need for oxygen, the myoglobin will quickly provide the oxygen. When the muscles are working hard and there is an immediate need for $O_2$, the myoglobin is there to supply it. It serves to take oxygen from the hemoglobin and act as a storage site for the molecule until it is needed. It would not work well as a transporter of oxygen from the lungs to the cells.

The difference between the percent saturation of myoglobin and that of hemoglobin at 40 mm reflects the results of the interaction of the heme-globin units with each other. Notice that the S-shaped Bohr curve is rather steep at 40 mm. This implies that any factors that shift the curve to the right or the left by even a small amount will have a significant effect on the quantity of oxygen that will be released in the capillaries. In Figure 24 are examples of shifted curves. The A curve is the normal Bohr curve. The B curve has been shifted to the right. Any shift of the Bohr curve to the right results in lower percent saturation at 40 mm. The hemoglobin molecule's affinity for oxygen is decreased by any factor that will shift the curve in this direction. As a result of this shift to the right, the lower percent saturation of oxygen, and the decrease in oxygen affinity, there is an increase in the amount of oxygen available to the cells.

## Figure 24. Shifts in the Bohr Curve

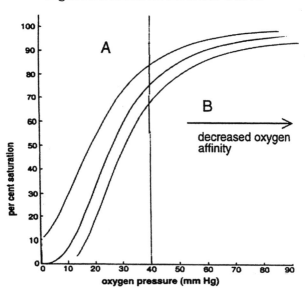

On the other hand, when the curve shifts to the left it intersects the 40 mm line at a higher percent saturation. Now the molecule's affinity for oxygen has increased, its percent saturation is higher, and it makes less oxygen available to the cells.

In the capillaries there is an increase in $CO_2$ pressure and in the amount of $CO_2$ dissolved in the blood. Increases in carbon dioxide concentration will shift the Bohr curve to the right. The $CO_2$ in the blood reacts with water to form carbonic acid ($H_2CO_3$) that ionizes to give hydrogen ions ($H^+$) and bicarbonate ions ($HCO_3^-$). Increases in $H^+$, which means an increase in acidity and a drop in pH[†], will also shift the curve to the right.

Thus, when there is more $CO_2$ and increased acidity in the blood, as in periods of high physical activity, the Bohr curve shifts to the right, the hemoglobin's affinity for oxygen decreases, and more oxygen is released to the cells. If acidity and carbon dioxide levels drop, the hemoglobin will hold on to oxygen with a greater affinity. In the lungs where $CO_2$ is lost, hemoglobin's affinity for oxygen increases. This relationship was discovered by Bohr, Hasselbach and King, but it is generally called the "Bohr effect." It appears that the most significant factor is the pH. While some carbon dioxide actually reacts with the hemoglobin molecule, the majority is transported in the plasma as bicarbonate ion with the corresponding $H^+$ held by the hemoglobin molecule.

One other important regulator of the Bohr effect is the concentration in the red cell of a molecule known as 2,3-DPG[†]. It is an organic phosphate present in very small concentrations in most cells, but every erythrocyte has such high levels that there is one 2,3-DPG molecule for each hemoglobin molecule. If the 2,3-DPG is removed from a red cell, hemoglobin's affinity for oxygen increases. (The Bohr curve moves to the left.) The 2,3-DPG molecule can react with specific sites on the hemoglobin molecule and discourage the formation of oxyhemoglobin. If 2,3-DPG is removed, it becomes easier for the oxygen to attach to the hemoglobin.

The 2,3-DPG is in the red cell as part of the pathway through which the cells obtain energy for glucose. While we have pictured the red cell as simply

---

† For those not familiar with the term, pH is a scale used to measure the acidity of a solution. It has nothing to do with pressure, as in pO2. The pH scale runs from 1 to 14. The lower the number, the greater the acidity.
† 2,3-diphosphoglycerate

a bag of hemoglobin, it is still a living cell and must keep up some metabolic functions. (Maintaining and repairing the cell membrane, for example.) This metabolic pathway is also dependent on the concentration of $H^+$. As the level of hydrogen ion increases the concentration of 2,3-DPG drops. This causes the Bohr curve to shift left to counteract the shift to the right due to the increase in acidity and carbonate ion.

It was noted in Chapter 1 that the fetus has a hemoglobin (Hb F) that differs slightly from that of its mother. The result of this difference is that the 2,3-DPG binds less tightly to the molecule and there is a slight shift to the left of the Bohr curve for Hb F as compared to that for Hb A. The fetal hemoglobin thus has a slightly higher affinity for oxygen than the maternal hemoglobin. This makes it possible for the baby to obtain oxygen from the mother when their bloods pass near each other in the placenta.

Finally, we should also observe that the body's temperature also alters the Bohr curve. At lower temperatures, when the oxygen demanded by the cells is lower, the curve shifts to the left. The hemoglobin has a greater affinity for the oxygen and less is available for the cells. In a fever, the increased temperature shifts the curve to the right. The blood can deliver more oxygen to meet the increased needs of the body for oxygen to fight the fever.

Understanding the way in which hemoglobin works also helps explain why some gases are poisonous. When carbon monoxide (CO), for example, enters the blood stream, it reacts readily with hemoglobin on the same site where oxygen binds. However, the CO forms such a strong bond with the iron that the reaction cannot be reversed. The product of this reaction, carbonmonoxyhemoglobin, can no longer transport oxygen. The oxygen carrying capacity of the blood is reduced. If carbon monoxide levels increase, the body suffers from the sudden onset of a rapidly developing anemia. The severity of the poisoning is in direct proportion to the amount of CO inhaled. Because carbon monoxide is colorless and odorless, an individual may become unconscious and die without ever becoming aware of having been exposed to the gas. Other poisons may impair the utilization of oxygen by the cells rather than the transport of oxygen to the cells. Alcohol, narcotics and poisons like cyanide prevent the cells from using oxygen even though there is an adequate supply.

Soon after people began to understand the circulation of blood and its role in the support of life, there was a interest in finding a material that can be used as a substitute for this critical fluid. Not long after the publication of Harvey's book, efforts were made to discover other liquids that could be used to replace blood or to find a way to transfer blood from one human to another. After three hundred years we have not found a substitute for this marvelous fluid, but we have developed techniques that make possible the routine collection, testing, storage, transport, and transfusion of human blood.

Unfortunately, outside the body blood is not very stable. Special chemicals must be added to it to prevent it from clotting into an unusable mass. Even then it is suitable for transfusion for only a few weeks. Relatively fresh supplies must always be available to handle emergencies. In addition, recent experiences with hepatitis and AIDS have created general concerns about the potential for transfer of pathogenic organisms during blood transfusions.

For these reasons work continues to find a stable, artificial substitute for blood. The military services are especially interested in this project. Unfortunately, there will  probably always be a need for a substance that can transport oxygen and replace fluids lost in battlefield wounds and trauma. It would also be advantageous to have a stable, safe replacement for blood needed during emergency and elective surgeries, for trauma victims, and for many types of treatment therapies.

The earliest efforts at finding a blood substitute involved the use of wines, beers, milk, or the blood of other animals. Richard Lower and Edmund King, in England, were probably the first to successfully transfer blood from one animal to another. They reported the results of their experiment to take blood from one dog and inject it into another in 1665. The first human transfusions into humans were performed in France in 1667 by Jean Baptiste Denis, physician to Louis XIV. Denis claimed to have saved a young boy's life by injecting him with a small amount of lamb's blood. His second patient also survived, but the third died. The procedure was not reliable, and the medical community generally lost interest in the idea until the 19th century. In 1818 James Blundell, an obstetrician, revived interest in the idea of blood transfusion. He managed to transfuse five patients safely with human blood. In the process he developed some useful techniques for conducting the procedure. However, there were still too many problems and too many failures. It was not possible to achieve consistent results. This is not surprising as there was no understanding of blood clotting and how to control it, no knowledge of bacterial infections and how to prevent them, and, most importantly, there was no realization that there is sometimes an incompatibility between one person's blood and any foreign cells that might be introduced into it, even cells from another person's blood.

The first two problems were solved by the end of the century. In 1835 T. Bischoff in Germany described the basics of blood clotting. Then Louis Pasteur's work on putrefaction and Joseph Lister's development of aseptic techniques to prevent contamination during medical procedures reduced the chances of infections during blood transfusion.

The third problem was not solved until the 20th century when Karl Landsteiner discovered blood groups. Dr. Landsteiner (1868-1943) was an immunologist who had been trained in medicine at the University of Vienna. In 1900 he published his first paper describing how the red blood cells of some people would clump, or agglutinate, when mixed with the blood of others. He studied these reactions for over 40 years and established the basic concepts of blood groups that we follow today. Landsteiner found that he could divide red cells into three groups: A, B, and O. (Later his assistants found a fourth group, AB.) Blood could be transfused into patients without agglutination only if it were from the appropriate blood group. Thus it is only necessary to "type" the blood from a donor and that of a recipient to make certain they are compatible. By 1921 all the major problems related to blood transfusions had been solved. This ability to collect, store, and transfuse human blood took away the pressure to find an artificial substitute.

However, work continued to develop blood replacements, and many different approaches have been tried. It is possible to make artificial solutions to replace the fluid volume and many of the components of blood, but nothing has been found to take the place of hemoglobin for transporting oxygen. Actually, the best replacement for a red cell filled with hemoglobin has, so far, been a solution of free hemoglobin. The use of free hemoglobin has a major problem in that the body has its own built-in mechanism for removing hemoglobin from the blood.

The body has a process established to remove aged red cells from the blood stream as it passes through the spleen, liver, bone marrow, or kidneys. The cell membrane is destroyed, the iron is recycled, the heme is degraded and excreted with the feces, and the globins are converted to free amino acids for reuse to the manufacture of other proteins. If there should be hemolysis (rupturing) of a red cell while circulating, hemoglobin molecules will be released into the blood. When this happens, the four-part hemoglobin molecule breaks apart into two dimers (with one alpha and one beta chain each). These dimers are picked up by other substances in the blood, primarily the haptoglobin molecule, and taken to the liver where they are destroyed. Excessive hemolysis of red cells will overload this hemoglobin removal system. Some of the dimers will be excreted in the urine (turning it red), and another serum protein, albumin, will help by binding to and removing the dimers. A solution of free hemoglobin could be transfused into a person who had lost a lot of blood. The free hemoglobin would transport oxygen, but the body would immediately make efforts to remove it.

There are some indications that hemoglobin must be removed from the blood because the molecule may be harmful to some of the tissues in the body. The kidneys seem to be especially sensitive to damage by an excess of free hemoglobin. However, there are also indications that it is not the hemoglobin itself that is toxic but other substances, like pieces of red cell membranes, that have been created or injected with the hemoglobin. Damage to tissues may have been the result of impurities that were injected with the hemoglobin solution.

The question of toxicity of hemoglobin is obviously important if we consider using solutions of free hemoglobin as a blood replacement. There are indications that hemoglobin molecules might be chemically modified to prevent their breakdown into dimers. The whole molecule is not so easily eliminated from the body and does not seem to have the possible toxic side effects that the dimer has. There are also efforts to use modified hemoglobins from other animals to produce blood substitutes.

# Chapter 5

# THE MAKING OF HEMOGLOBIN

This sophisticated and complex molecule so well suited for gas transport is continuously manufactured in the human body. Each second the average adult produces over 20 million red cells, and each of these red cells contains approximately 300 million molecules of hemoglobin. Twenty different amino acids are the raw materials from which the red cell must assemble alpha and beta chains. And when these amino acids are linked together, it is critical that they be unerringly combined in a specific sequence. One error in the selection of a single amino acid, as occurs in the formation of hemoglobin S, can create problems for the body. After manufacturing the globin chains the red cell must make heme, put an iron in the center, combine one heme molecule with one globin chain, then join four heme-globin units to form the final hemoglobin molecule.

The same process is repeated over and over, day after day, billions upon billions of times during the life of each individual.

It all starts in the bone marrow.

When asked to name the organs in the body, few people think of the bone marrow. Yet, it is, in fact, the largest organ (by weight) in the human body. The total weight of the bone marrow in a typical adult is between 1.5 and 3.0 kilograms (3.3 – 6.6 lbs.). The marrow is a tissue located in a cavity that extends through the inside of bones. Half this tissue is yellow, fatty, and inactive. The remainder, known as red stroma or reticulum, is the site of production of all red cells, some white cells, and platelets.

The reticulum of the bone marrow produces a continual supply of small cells called "stem" cells. These cells sit idle in the bone marrow until each one receives a chemical message telling it to become a platelet, a white cell, or a red cell. The platelets flow through the blood stream until needed to form a clot to prevent the escape of blood from a vessel wall. The white cells are active agents in the immune system and aid in the body's fight against infection. The red cells, of course, are needed for gas transport.

**Figure 25. Red Blood Cell Production**

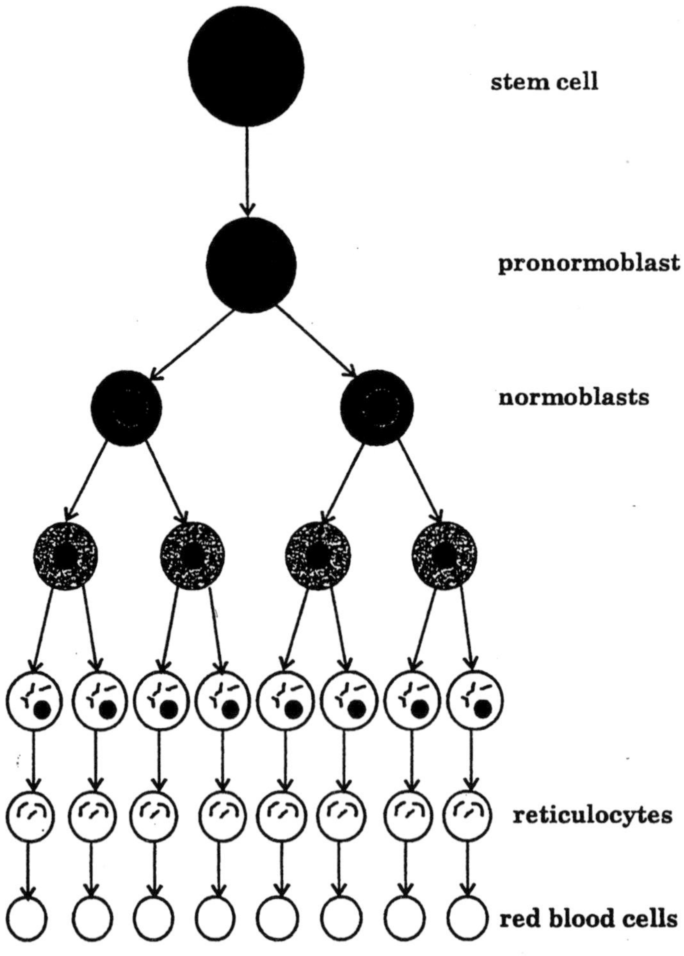

The technical name for red blood cells is erythrocytes, and the process by which the red cells are formed is called erythropoiesis. It does not occur in every bone in the body but is limited primarily to the ends of long bones, the sternum, ribs, skull, vertebrae, and the large flat bones in the pelvis. The chemical signal that starts the stem cell on the path to becoming a red cell is actually produced in the kidneys.

If the supply of oxygen arriving at the kidney tissues starts to drop off, the cells will secrete REF (renal erythropoietin factor). The REF, in turn, converts a substance in the blood plasma to erythropoietin (EPO). The blood carries the erythropoietin through the body with it until it eventually passes through the bone marrow. There it reacts with a stem cell and initiates its conversion to an erythrocyte. As more red cells are produced, the supply of oxygen to the kidneys increases, the production of REF declines, the amount of EPO in the blood decreases, and the creation of new red cells slows down. Thus the body has a feedback mechanism for producing red cells in response to its need for oxygen.

A stem cell that has just started on its way to becoming an erythrocyte is called a pronormoblast. It divides three times in the next 3-4 days, and from one pronormoblast come eight normoblasts. (See Figure 25.) It is in these normoblasts (still in the bone marrow) that the production of hemoglobin takes place. To understand how the normoblast is able to accurately produce millions of hemoglobin molecules in just a few seconds is to understand the answer to one of the basic questions of life: how does a living organism know how to make the proteins it needs?

Each individual starts life with a set of blueprints. These blueprints are in the form of a code carried by the DNA molecule that forms the chromosomes. This DNA molecule consists of a backbone of sugar and phosphate molecules that are alternately attached to each other in a long line. (See Figure 26.) Attached to each sugar molecule is one of only four specific molecules called bases. These bases belong to a group of organic compounds known as nucleotides. There are only four found in DNA, and these four carry the entire genetic code. They are adenine, guanine, cytosine, and thymine. They are most often referred to by their first letters alone: A, G, C, and T. The genetic code that we each inherit is in the form of a long string to which are attached, in a specific sequence, G, C, A and T. Each group of three bases, called a codon, specifies a particular amino acid. For example, GGG indicates glycine, CAC is histidine, etc.

## Figure 26. Structure of DNA

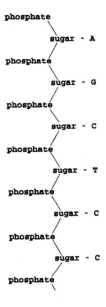

In the normoblast there is a nucleus with 23 pairs of chromosomes – half of each pair comes from the father, half from the mother. These chromosome pairs do not look alike. When viewed through a microscope, they each have a distinctive size and shape. They have been identified by numbering them from 1 to 22. The final pair, which determines the sex of the person, is either XX (female) or XY (male). On chromosome number 11 there is a segment of the DNA molecule that tells the cell the exact sequence of amino acids needed to make a beta chain. On chromosome 16 are other segments that carry the code for the alpha chain.

Once the normoblast has been informed that it is ready to start making hemoglobin, it must translate the code into a real protein. First it <u>transcribes</u> the code from the DNA molecule to a similar molecule called RNA. The code in the DNA segment that carries the information needed to make a protein is used to make an RNA with the same information. In RNA, however, the thymine (T) is replaced with uracil (U) and the four nucleotide bases in RNA are not CGAT, but CGAU. And, to further complicate matters, each base is transcribed, not as itself but as a complementary base. The bases are complementary because their structures are such that they form strong bonds when placed next to each other. Thus, G and C are complements of each other;

likewise, A and T (or U, in the case of RNA). The G on DNA becomes a C on RNA, C becomes G, A would be a T but is a U, instead, and T becomes A.

This DNA code:      -G-G-G-C-A-T-T-A-A-A-C-C-A-T-
is transcribed to
this RNA code:      -C-C-C-G-U-A-A-U-U-U-G-G-U-A-

The RNA segment now leaves the nucleus of the cells, where the chromosomes are located, and enters the cell's cytoplasm. One strand of RNA carrying the genetic code for one particular protein chain is called a messenger RNA (or mRNA). It attaches itself to a ribosome floating in the cytoplasm.

It is on the ribosome that the coded message carried by the mRNA is translated into the formation of a protein. Also floating around in the cytoplasm are small, hairpin-shaped molecules called transfer RNA (or tRNA). There is one specific tRNA molecule for each amino acid. At the bottom, curved end of the hairpin are three bases, the anticodon. Attached to the top of the hairpin is one amino acid – the specific amino acid coded by the complement of the sequence of three bases at the other end of the molecule. (Figure 27.)

As each mRNA passes through the ribosome, each codon, or set of 3 bases, in order, becomes attached to the corresponding anticodon on a tRNA. The amino acids on the ends of the tRNA's, as they are lined up in the correct sequence, are linked together to form the protein. The amino acids separate from the tRNA, and the used tRNA returns to the cytoplasm to pick up another amino acid. Meanwhile, the mRNA continues to pass through the ribosome, and the next 3-base code is read. (Figure 28.)

## Figure 27. Transfer RNA

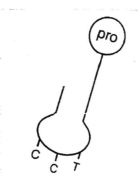

To better understand the process, we can follow the trail of one particular amino acid in one particular protein. The beta chain of hemoglobin A starts with the following eight amino acids:

Val-his-leu-thr-pro-glu-glu-lys-
 1   2   3   4   5   6   7   8

The DNA code for the sixth amino acid, glutamic acid, is GAG. When the mRNA is formed, the G becomes C and A becomes U. Thus the RNA code reads CUC. In the ribosome, the CUC on the mRNA reacts with the anticodon GAG on a transfer RNA. At the other end of the tRNA molecule is glutamic acid (glu). When the time comes in the process of synthesizing the protein, glu is placed in the sixth position of the beta chain of the hemoglobin molecule.

If there were an error in the DNA code and the GAG had been replaced by GTG, the result would be different. The new mRNA code would be CAC, the corresponding tRNA anticodon would be GTG, which is the code for valine (val). As a result of this one change in the nucleotide sequence, the sixth amino acid would be valine, not glutamic acid. This is, in fact, what happens in sickle-cell anemia. The Hb S beta chain starts with:

Val-his-leu-thr-pro-val-glu-lys-
 1   2   3   4   5   6   7   8

There are, of course, many other complications in the normal process of reading the DNA code and producing a protein. There are codes that regulate the rate at which a protein is made. Codes are present that indicate where on the DNA molecule a specific protein code starts and stops. All of these activities are aided by many enzymes that assist and speed up the reactions. These enzymes are coded in other sections of the DNA. Even with all these complications, there are still large segments of DNA that carry information that is of no apparent use to our bodies.

**Figure 28. The Synthesis of a Protein**

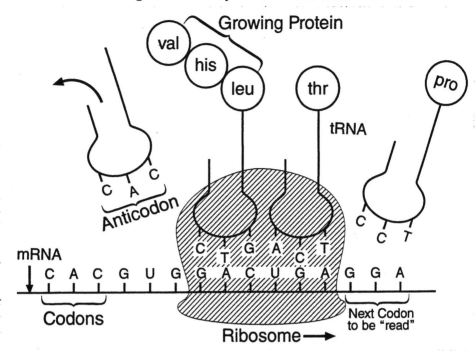

The information for manufacturing the hemoglobin alpha chains is found on chromosome 16. That for the beta is on chromosome 11. Because the heme is not a protein, there isn't a specific section of the DNA code for it. Instead, the cell makes a series of enzymes that carry out a sequence of reactions that result in a heme molecule.

The synthesis of proteins like the globin chains occurs in the ribosomes of the normoblasts. The production of heme takes place in the mitochondrion – a separate part of the normoblast. There, enzymes are produced that are responsible for the catalysis of a sequence of reactions. The result of these reactions is the formation of a complete heme. A generalized scheme of this series of reactions is presented in Figure 29. The process starts when the enzyme ALA synthetase forms delta-aminolevulinic acid (ALA) from the amino acid glycine and a molecule of succinic acid. Each of the ALA molecules contains 5 carbon atoms and a nitrogen. Two ALA molecules are combined to form a circular molecule known as porphobilinogen.

Next, four porphobilinogen molecules are joined together to create protoporphyrin, which undergoes some slight modification to become porphyrin. All that is lacking at this point is iron. Transferrin molecules in the blood pick up iron atoms and carry them to the bone marrow. Each normoblast has a special receptor on its surface where transferrin can attach itself. While bound to the cell, the transferrin gives up its iron atom to the cellular molecule apoferritin. The apoferritin-iron reaction produces ferritin – a granular storage for iron that is used up as heme is produced. Finally, the enzyme heme synthetase inserts an iron atom into each porphyrin molecule to complete the formation of heme.

The heme molecules are combined with globin molecules sometime during their production. It is not known for certain exactly when this happens. Finally, two alpha-heme units and two beta-heme units are joined to form the final hemoglobin molecule.

As the concentration of hemoglobin in the normoblast increases, the size of the nucleus shrinks. Finally, the production of hemoglobin stops and the nucleus disappears. The resulting cell is called a reticulocyte.

The reticulocyte stage, which lasts about 48 hours, represents the final step in the conversion of a stem cell to a mature red cell. It is now ready for work. There are small blood vessels passing through the bone marrow, and as the reticulocyte squeezes through the vascular wall any remaining nuclear material is trapped and held back. In humans the erythrocyte that enters the blood stream has no nuclear material and is not able to synthesize hemoglobin. It not only loses its nuclear material, but the ribosomes, where the globins were made, and the mitochondria, where heme was created, have also disappeared. In reptiles and birds the circulating red cells still have the nuclear material.

**Figure 29. The Production of Heme**

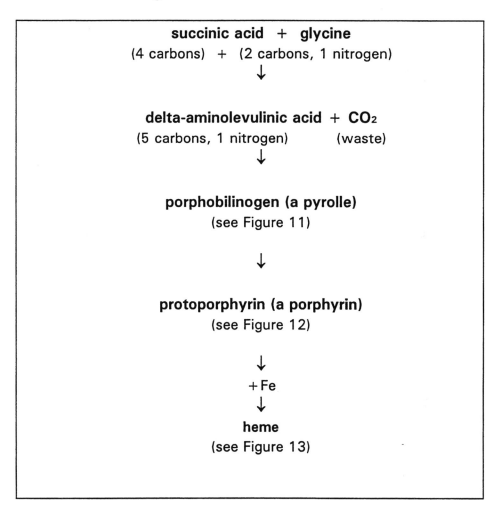

In their travels through the body the red cells pass through the spleen. This organ, about the size of an adult's fist, is directly beneath the diaphragm just behind and to the left of the stomach. The spleen produces lymphocytes and takes an active part in the body's defenses against infections. One of its other functions is to remove the "rubbish" in the red cells. This rubbish can come from several sources. Remnants of nuclear material left over in the cell and material that was not combed out by the vascular wall in the bone marrow will form small particles, called Howell-Jolly bodies, in the red cell. If the red cell had taken in more iron than was needed for heme production, small deposits called siderotic granules may form. Sometimes, usually as a result of a genetic disorder, some hemoglobin molecules will denature (a process similar to the hardening of an egg white in hot water) and form particles known as Heinz bodies.

All of these materials are removed by the spleen. As the cells pass through the spleen they must squeeze through minute pores 1-2 µm in size. The normal red cell is very flexible and easily deforms to pass through the small opening. The solid, non-compressible inclusions (the Howell-Jolly bodies, the siderotic granules, and the Heinz bodies) will not pass through. They are trapped in the spleen and pinched off. Thus the spleen grooms and cleans the red cells, improving their life and efficiency. This process has been compared to what happens when a dog passes through a spring door. The dog can squeeze through, but his tail is caught by the door as the spring pulls it shut.

It is also in the spleen where the aged red cells are destroyed. In the course of its 120-day life each red cell travels approximately 200 miles. During that time it is subjected to repeat compression and decompression as it squeezes in and out of capillaries and general wear and tear as it passes through the blood vessels. Although the exact chemical changes that reflect this aging process are unknown, it is apparent that the spleen has some way to spot and destroy these older cells.

The actual destruction of the aged red cells is done by *macrophages*, large cells produced by the spleen. Macrophages are also produced by the lymphatic system and used to destroy bacteria during an infection. In fact, during an infection the rate of formation of macrophages can become so great that the lymph nodes enlarge and become tender. If the spleen should happen to be removed from an individual, the process of red cell destruction can still be accomplished by the macrophages in the lymph system.

After the red cells are destroyed the hemoglobin molecules are degraded. The globin chains are converted back into the basic amino acids, which are returned to the body's pool of amino acids. The iron molecule is saved by attaching it to the molecule transferrin in the plasma for reuse. The heme molecules (without the iron) become bilirubin, which is carried to the liver, formed into bile, and excreted into the intestines.

There is one additional complication. So far we have talked about hemoglobin as if there were only one normal hemoglobin. There are, in fact, several normal components of hemoglobin. Between conception and birth the developing human fetus produces several different hemoglobins. Even the hemoglobin molecules in the normal adult do not all have the same structure. These hemoglobins differ from each other in the exact sequences of amino acids in the globin chains. While the heme molecules are all the same, the globin chains are different. Each time the genes create a different sequence of amino acids for the globin chain the chain is given a different name by using a different letter of the Greek alphabet.

The single cell that starts each human life contains all the genetic information needed for that cell to develop into an embryo, a fetus, a baby, a child and, finally, an adult. As the single starting cell divides and proliferates into other cells it passes all the genetic information it has to every cell. Yet, as the organism grows the cells begin to specialize. Soon each cell only uses a small part of that information it has inherited. Brain cells do not use the same information that liver cells need. Red cells only need the information used to produce hemoglobin and a few other substances. The muscle cells have their own needs and make no use of the genetic details on the manufacture of hemoglobin.

During the embryonic and fetal stages much of the genetic information is needed to promote the growth and development of the body. As the organism reaches each stage in its development, the appropriate DNA information is used to grow to the next. When no longer needed, the genetic information is turned off. The code is still there, but it is somehow blocked off and not read by the cells.

Despite this need for all these changes and cell specializations, there is still a great deal of genetic information that remains unused. Some of it appears to be genetic information left from an evolutionary past, other parts of the DNA molecule seem to be meaningless, although it is possible that we simply don't understand its purpose. In addition to the information for making the proteins, the DNA contains details that tell where proteins start and stop, that promote the formation of proteins when needed, and so on.

In the very early stages of embryonic development, during the first three weeks of life, the cells start to differentiate into three basic groups: the ectoderm, which will cover the embryo and develop into skin, hair, tooth enamel, etc.; the endoderm, which lines the premature gut; and the mesoderm, which lies between the other two. The mesoderm will develop into the circulatory system, blood cells, muscles, ligaments, and connective tissue.

Late in the third week of life some of the cells in the mesoderm form clusters called blood islands. The cells around the outside of these islands eventually flatten and join together to form tubes of a vascular system. Some of the cells on the inside of these blood islands become the first hemoglobin-synthesizing cells.

The hemoglobins produced in this early stage do not have the same globin chains with the same amino acid sequences as the adult. The heme molecules are the same, but the embryonic globin chains are not like those in Hb A. The earliest hemoglobin consists of two zeta ($\zeta$) chains and two epsilon ($\in$) chains[27]. The zeta chain is a precursor of the alpha chain and, in fact, the genetic information for producing zeta chains is located on the same chromosome 16 near the DNA sequences that code for alpha chains. In a like manner, the epsilon chain is coded on chromosome 11 near that of the beta chain. This embryonic hemoglobin has been named Hb Gower-1 and its formula written as ($\zeta_2\in_2$).

## Figure 30. Human Globin Chains

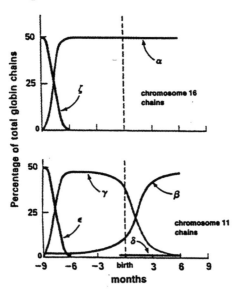

27 E. R. Huehns, N. Dance, G. H. Beaven, F. Hecht, and A. G. Motulsky, "Human embryonic hemoglobins," *Cold Spring Harbor Symp Quant Biol* 29: 327-331, 1969.

During its development the organism does not abruptly stop making one hemoglobin and switch to another. There is always a period of transition. However, each stable hemoglobin always contains two pairs of globin chains. (Figure 30.) One pair is alpha or a similar globin; the other pair is beta or a beta-like globin. Alpha chain production starts very early in life and its only precursor appears to be the zeta chain. Before eight weeks of life have passed the embryo has started to produce alpha chains. This results in the presence of Hb Gower-2 ($\alpha_2 \in_2$) along side the Hb Gower-1.

The epsilon chain is soon replaced by another $\beta$-like chain designated gamma ($\gamma$). In the early stages this results in the production of some Hb Portland ($\zeta_2 \gamma_2$). However, by the end of the seventh week after conception the major hemoglobin contains two alpha and two gamma chains. It is designated Hb F and remains the primary hemoglobin of the fetus. By the ninth week 90% of the hemoglobin is Hb F.

During the sixth week of embryonic life the production of the beta chain begins. This means there will be a small amount of Hb A ($\alpha_2 \beta_2$) in the early stages of fetal development, but the level of Hb A increases very slowly and there is not a significant switch from gamma chain production to beta chain production until the 30th week. At birth the gamma chain synthesis stops and beta chain production goes into full operation.

The actual levels of F and A in newborns vary from individual to individual, but there is typically 5-20% Hb A at birth. By the end of the first year after birth Hb A is the major hemoglobin and typically constitutes 95-97% of the total hemoglobin in the child and the adult.

What is the other 3-5%? First, adults do not lose the ability to make Hb F; the process is simply turned off when we are born. However, it is not unusual for the adult to continue to make a small amount of Hb F, and levels of 0-1% Hb F in an adult are not unusual. In addition, there is also another hemoglobin component found in normal individuals that is different from hemoglobin A. This hemoglobin, designated Hb $A_2$, contains two alpha chains and two delta ($\delta$) chains. The delta chains are also coded on chromosome 11, along with the epsilon, gamma and beta chains. They contain the same number of amino acids as beta chains but differ from beta chains in amino acid sequence in ten places. Production of delta chains may start just before birth, but it never reaches very high levels. A typical adult might have only 1.5-2.5% Hb $A_2$ in the blood. Hb $A_2$ does not seem to have any particular function, and its presence may just be a reflection of an evolutionary past. The delta globin chain may have been used and discarded in one of the past stages of human evolution. However, for some reason its production has not been switched off completely and there are still traces in the body. While Hb $A_2$ in itself is neither good nor bad, its concentration can be used for certain diagnostic purposes. This will be discussed in greater detail in Chapter 7.

# Chapter 6

# ANEMIA

The measurement of total hemoglobin is the best single indicator of an individual's state of health. If physicians could have only one diagnostic test to perform on every person, they would obtain the greatest information about an individual's state of health by measuring the concentration of hemoglobin in the blood. In the United States there is a program to improve the health of lower income women and their young children. The WIC (women, infants and children) program, carried out by the Dept. of Agriculture, spends over 2 billion dollars a year to test and improve the nutritional state of young children, infants and expectant mothers. To monitor the general state of health and nutrition of the people they see, the WIC field service people.perform one test in the field — they measure total hemoglobin.

To measure the total hemoglobin of an individual it is necessary to use only a few drops of blood. The blood is mixed with a chemical that attacks and ruptures the red cell membrane. This process is called *lysing* the red cells and is necessary in order to free the hemoglobin.

A solution produced in this manner (i.e., by lysing red cells) is called an hemolysate. The hemolysate is then placed in an instrument that measures the amount of light absorbed by the solution. (As was noted by Felix Hoppe-Seyler, hemoglobin absorbs light at specific wavelengths.) The greater the absorption of light, the higher the concentration of hemoglobin in the blood.

A second, commonly used but indirect, way to determine total hemoglobin is to measure the hematocrit. A long glass capillary tube is used to collect a few drops of blood from a finger prick. The capillary tube is sealed at one end and placed in a centrifuge. Spinning the tube at high speeds causes the red cells to settle to the bottom of the tube. The hematocrit is the percentage of the total blood volume occupied by the red cells. (See Figure 31.)

Hemoglobin concentrations are reported as grams per 100 mL of blood. Since 100 mL is one tenth of a liter, or one deciliter (dL), the unit is grams/deciliter, or g/dL. Typical values for healthy individuals are given in Table II.

It has been generally observed that the hematocrit (in %) is approximately three times the hemoglobin concentration (in g/dL), and many people use this relationship to convert from one measure to the other (i.e., an hematocrit of 39% implies a hemoglobin concentration of 13 g/dL).

Anemia occurs when there is a reduction in the concentration of hemoglobin in the blood. Anemia is not a disease, it is the symptom of a disease or disorder. The decrease may be due to many reasons. Anemias may be caused by nutritional deficiencies that lead to inadequate red cell production, by abnormal bone marrow function, by accelerated destruction of red cells, by genetic conditions affecting the production of hemoglobin, or by excessive loss of blood.

## Figure 31. The Hematocrit

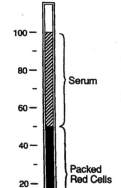

## Table II. Normal Hemoglobin Levels

| Group | Hemoglobin Concentration | Hematocrit |
|---|---|---|
| Males | 14 - 18 g/dL | 42 - 54 |
| Females | 12 - 16 g/dL | 36 - 48 |

The exact symptoms of a person with anemia as well as their frequency and severity will depend on the cause of the problem. Some individuals with a mild anemia may not have any particular symptoms other than occasional fatigue, palpitations of the heart, and difficulty "catching their breath" after exercising. Anemia can develop slowly in individuals with an internal bleeding problem (e.g., a bleeding ulcer) where the constant loss of small amounts of blood gradually lowers their hemoglobin level.

As the concentration of hemoglobin drops the heart starts to beat faster to increase the rate at which blood flows through the body. These palpitations are particularly noticeable after some muscular exertion when there is an increased need for oxygen. When hemoglobin levels drop below 7-8 g/dL, these palpitations are felt even when the body is at rest.

Other signs of anemia include dizziness, headaches, or ringing in the ears. Skin pallor has historically been a physical symptom associated with anemia, but it is not a good diagnostic indicator. Too many factors can alter the flow of blood to the skin, and there is too great a variation in skin pigmentation among humans.

The most common causes of anemia are nutritional disorders. In order to grow, divide, and multiply, the precursors of red blood cells need amino acids, minerals (e.g., iron, copper, and cobalt), and several enzymes (folic acid, vitamin $B_{12}$, riboflavin, nicotinic acid, pyridoxine, ascorbic acid, pantothenic acid, thiamine, choline, and biotin). Because red cells are produced so rapidly and in such large quantities, their production is often the first place the body reveals the existence of nutritional deficiencies. The most common cause of anemia in adults is the result of an iron deficiency when there is a depletion of iron stores needed to produce hemoglobin. This can occur when there is an increased demand for iron during periods of rapid growth in infants and children, and during pregnancy, when the growing fetus relies on the maternal stores of iron. It also occurs when there is significant blood loss and the body cannot produce the needed hemoglobin from its normal iron stores. This happens frequently in people with peptic ulcers, gastrointestinal tumors, and hemorrhoids. It can also be the result of malabsorption of nutrients into the body, the best known example being pernicious anemia.

While seen in all ages and races, pernicious anemia is predominantly a disease of the white race with particularly high incidence among Scandinavians, English, and Irish. It is very rare in Orientals. It is a disease mainly of late adult life and usually does not occur before age 40. The typical patients complain of not feeling up to par for the last few months. They seem to lack strength and energy. There is a feeling of general malaise. Their skin is pale, and they have trouble catching their breath after any kind of exertion. It can also be accompanied by other side effects: stomach upset, alternating constipation and diarrhea, and neurological complaints. Before the advances of modern medicine, pernicious anemia was frequently fatal.

In the last half of the 19th century it was noted that pernicious anemia was associated with some defect in the mucous membranes lining the stomach. In 1855 Addison described the disease and observed that is was accompanied by a decrease in the production of gastric juices. In 1870 Fenwick found that the mucous membrane from the stomach of a person with pernicious anemia could not attack the white of a hard-boiled egg. Attempts were made in research with dogs to discover if any foods could be given to counteract this problem. They found that liver had the greatest effect.

George Minot and William Murphy discovered in the 1920s that feeding large amounts of liver ( 1/2 lb of lightly cooked or raw liver per day) would improve the health of a patient with pernicious anemia. Dr. William Castle postulated that there was some nutrient (an extrinsic factor) in food which could not be absorbed into the stomach because of some other missing compound (an intrinsic factor) in the mucous membrane of the stomach.

It took 20 years of research, but by 1948 the extrinsic factor had been isolated from liver. It was found to be a large molecule with a cobalt atom in the center of a ring system similar to that of heme. The molecule was designated vitamin $B_{12}$ and was found only in animal foods (liver, meat, fish, and eggs). It wasn't until 1964 that the exact function of vitamin $B_{12}$ in the production of red cells was determined. It is needed to produce an enzyme that makes synthesis of DNA possible. Without production of DNA there can be no cell division. A lack of vitamin $B_{12}$ prevents the formation of new red cells in the bone marrow.

The intrinsic factor was found to be a glycoprotein molecule (i.e., a protein with a glucose attached to it) produced in the mucous membrane in the stomach and secreted with the gastric juices. This glycoprotein attaches itself to the $B_{12}$ molecule and forms a complex that can be absorbed into the body through the small intestine. The body cannot produce vitamin $B_{12}$ and must obtain it through diet. However, it can store $B_{12}$ in the liver. When there is a problem with the production of the intrinsic factor, it takes a while for the body to use up its stored reserves of $B_{12}$ before pernicious anemia starts to develop.

Other nutritional deficiencies can lead to reduced red cell production. The most common type of anemia in the world today is that caused by an iron deficiency. This occurs when there is too little iron taken into the body, usually as a result of a long period of starvation or poor diet. Someone with chronic diarrhea will have trouble absorbing iron from food because it does not stay in the small intestine long enough. During pregnancy the mother has increased iron needs because her body must provide iron for the developing fetus. An estimated one billion people in the world are anemic because they have low iron levels. The WIC program, mentioned previously, was created in the 1970s to deal with the problem of iron deficiency in the U.S. It is administered by the Department of Agriculture and involves the distribution of free food to economically disadvantaged people most at risk for nutritional deficiencies: pregnant women, children from birth to age 5, and lactating women. Infants receive iron-fortified formula; children and women are provided with iron-fortified cereals, vitamin C-fortified juices, eggs, milk, and other nutritional foods to enrich their diets. Studies have indicated the program has worked and there has been a significant decrease in the number of people in the targeted group who suffer from anemia[28].

In addition to vitamin $B_{12}$ deficiency, a lack of folic acid in the diet will lead to reduced red cell production. Folic acid is a vitamin also needed for the growth and division of cells. There are three groups of people at greatest risk

[28] J. A. Stockman, "Iron Deficiency Anemia: Have We Come Far Enough?," *JAMA* 258(12):1645-1647, Sept. 25, 1987.

for anemia due to decreased levels of folic acid: pregnant women, people over the age of 50, and chronic alcoholics. During pregnancy a women may need double the normal amount of folic acid to satisfy her needs as well as those of the fetus. In the elderly there is a danger of folic acid deficiency when the diet lacks fresh fruit and vegetables — excellent sources of folic acid. Alcoholics may be in danger because of a poor diet and the interference of alcohol in the process of absorption of the folic acid into the body.

Aplastic anemias are those caused by failure of the bone marrow to produce adequate numbers of red cells. In 50% of the cases of aplastic anemia the exact cause is unknown. In the remainder it is due to some toxic substance to which the individual is particularly sensitive. Cancer patients undergoing treatment with radiation and chemotherapy can also suffer from an aplastic anemia.

Anemia can be caused by errors in the production of the hemoglobin in the red cell. When the disorder is related to the globins, it is a 'hemoglobinopathy.' If there is a genetically caused reduction in the manufacture of one of the globin chains, it is called a thalassemia. They will be discussed in greater detail in the next chapter. On the other hand, there can also be production of abnormal hemoglobin variants, and these conditions will be covered in chapter 8. We have already seen how one variant, Hb S, can cause sickle-cell disease. The sickling of the cells decreases their life span and their ability to bring oxygen to the cells of the body. The result is an anemia.

A condition in which there is destruction of the red cells in the blood is called a hemolytic anemia. Hemolytic anemia may either be acquired by a person (caused by some external factor), or it may be the result of heredity, or it may be a combination of both factors. The lysing of the red cells will dump hemoglobin molecules in the blood stream. The kidneys will attempt to remove the hemoglobin and, as a result, the urine will turn red.

In the 6th century B.C. Pythagoras, the Greek philosopher and mathematician, set up a school near Crotona, in southern Italy. For the students who came to study under him Pythagoras established rules that turned the school into a monastic community of scholars. All goods were held in common, and there were very strict rules that had to be obeyed. The followers of Pythagoras were forbidden to eat meat, eggs, or beans. Tradition reports that Pythagoras' aversion to beans was so strong that his followers were not even allowed to walk through a field of beans! There is also a story that

Pythagoras refused to enter a bean field to save his own life. He was being pursued by a mob of townspeople who resented his attempts to interfere with local government. They chased him to the edge of a bean field, which he refused to enter. As a result, he was caught and slain.

Pythagoras' dislike of beans may seem arbitrary and unreasonable, or some might attribute it to a concern for excessive flatulence, but 25 centuries later scientists may have found a very valid reason for it. For centuries in many villages throughout the Mediterranean countries it was observed that every February a significant number of people, both youths and adults, would start to feel lethargic. They complained of dizziness and nausea. They would fall asleep easily and lacked the energy to do any work. For most the problem would last about three months, and they would recover. A few would start to pass blood in their urine, and some of the more severe cases would die. In Sardinia as many as 35% of the people in some villages suffered from this malady.

Their anemia is caused by the loss of hemoglobin as a result of the lysing of red blood cells. In more serious cases the urine turns red as the free hemoglobin in the blood is removed in the kidneys. In the 1950s scientists discovered that there is a very high incidence of G-6-PD deficiency in this population. G-6-PD (short for glucose-6-phosphate dehydrogenase) is an enzyme in the red blood cells that takes part in some of the chemical reactions needed to produce energy for the cell to operate. Those people who inherited G-6-PD deficiency would suffer from this seasonal hemolytic anemia. Since they did not suffer all year round, there must be something in their environment that triggered the disease.

They found the answer in the beans. The fava, or Italian broad, bean is very prolific in Mediterranean countries. It is grown in abundance and is a staple for the local populations during the spring and summer. For many it is an important, tasty, and nutritious addition to their diet. However, those with G-6-PD deficiency who eat uncooked, or lightly cooked, fava beans, or who breath in the pollen of fava bean plants, can suffer from hemolytic anemia. Some compound in the beans appears to interfere with the metabolism of the red cells. For some reason the cells clump together and lyse. Normal individuals, who have G-6-PD, have a mechanism for neutralizing the adverse effect of the fava beans.

In may be that Pythagoras had G-6-PD deficiency and noted that eating fava beans or breathing the pollen made him ill. He would not allow his followers to eat beans, probably assuming that it could cause a similar illness in others. The world would have to wait 2,500 years to find the scientific basis for his fear of beans.

Hemolytic anemia is also reported frequently as an adverse reaction to some drugs. In 1926 pamaquine, a drug used very effectively to treat malaria, was found to cause hemolytic anemia in 4 out of 36 blacks to whom it had been given. This was not particularly unusual; many drugs are known to cause hemolytic anemia. Researchers assumed the drug was toxic to a certain number of individuals and, even though a good antimalarial, ignored its uses because of its toxic properties.

Additional research found that one out of ten blacks are susceptible to another antimalarial drug, primaquine. This problem was found to occur in people with G-6-PD deficiency. Individuals who inherit a reduced ability to produce G-6-PD may not suffer any particular problem until their blood is exposed to some agent that will produce hemolytic anemia when there is a deficiency of this enzyme. The exact mechanism is not completely understood, but about 100 million people in the world, including three million in the U.S., have G-6-PD deficiency.

Some individuals acquire autoimmune diseases in which they start to destroy their own red cells at an increased rate. This hemolytic anemia is often secondary to the major problem, but it seems to complicate the course of the disorder and its treatment. Often the autoimmune response is triggered by a medication that causes the body to destroy its own red cells. Drugs that have been known to cause autoimmune disease include antibiotics (penicillin, tetracycline, and streptomycin), a compound that lowers blood pressure (methyldopa), and a sedative (chlorpromazine).

Those who believe they are suffering from an anemia should seek the help of a physician to determine the underlying cause. Taking vitamins and iron pills may help, but there may be a more serious problem that should be investigated as soon as possible. There are even a few situations where the extra iron would make the problem worse. In iron-overload anemia (also known as sideroblastic anemia) the red cells cannot use the iron effectively in forming the hemoglobin molecule. Excess iron accumulates in the bone marrow and the liver, and taking extra iron only adds to these deposits.

It is best to find the cause of the anemia and directly treat the source of the problem.

# Chapter 7

# ANEMIAS OF THE SEA

It was noted in the last chapter that anemia is a symptom, not a disease in itself, and that it can be caused by several different factors. One particular group of anemias, known as thalassemias, result when there is reduced production of one of the globin chains needed to manufacture hemoglobin. The developing red cell should ideally produce equal numbers of alpha (or alpha-like) globin chains and beta (or beta-like) globins. In the normal red cell there should be just enough alpha to react with all the beta, delta and gamma chains present to produce Hb A, Hb F, and Hb A$_2$. If, however, there is some condition that causes the cell to underproduce one chain with respect to its corresponding complement, there will be fewer hemoglobin molecules produced. This leaves the red cell with an excess of one globin chain, less hemoglobin than it should have, and a reduced capacity for transporting oxygen.

Since there can be a corresponding thalassemia associated with each globin chain, the specific condition is described by prefixing the word *thalassemia* with the name of the chain involved. The most common thalassemias are naturally alpha and beta. While gamma-, epsilon-, delta-, and zeta-thalassemias are known to exist, they have not been studied in great detail.

Thalassemias appear to be the most common inherited disorder of the human race. There must have been thousands of people with thalassemia seen by physicians before the disease was specifically named and distinguished as a separate disorder. Credit for first describing thalassemias goes to a Detroit physician, Dr. Thomas Cooley. He was originally from Ann Arbor, Michigan, graduated in medicine in 1895, and studied in Boston and Germany. He practiced medicine in Detroit and eventually worked full-time at the Children's Hospital there. In 1925 Dr. Cooley and his collaborator, Dr. Pearl Lee, published an article in the *Transactions of the American Pediatric Society*[29]. They described four children with anemia, enlargement of the spleen and liver, discoloration of the skin and the sclerae, and no bile in the urine. These children also had a Mongoloid appearance caused by enlargement of the cranial and facial bones.

Over the next few years similar cases were described in North American and European medical literature. It was noted that the disease seemed to be particularly prevalent among people who came from countries surrounding the Mediterranean Sea. Italian and Greek investigators began describing a high incidence of the disorder in their countries. Early reports referred to the condition as Cooley's anemia or Mediterranean anemia.

In 1936 Whipple and Bradford, two physicians in Rochester NY, published a paper[30] on the disease and gave it the name 'thalassemia.' The word came from the Greek word for sea (thalassa), and Dr. Whipple felt this term would retain the association of the condition with peoples from the Mediterranean.

Dr. Caminoptros, a Greek physician, was the first to propose in 1936 that the disease was hereditary. This conclusion was supported by the work of several investigators in Italy and the United States. By 1949 it was well accepted that thalassemia is an inherited disorder, but there was still much confusion because of the highly variable nature of the disease. In most genetic disorders we expect to find two separate and distinct states: the heterozygous, where the individual carries the trait but still has one normal gene, and the homozygous, where both genes are defective. The thalassemias, in contrast, appeared to come in a multiplicity of forms and conditions ranging from fairly mild to extremely severe.

The first clues as to the genetic problem that causes thalassemia came from studies of an individual who had inherited both sickle-cell trait and

---

29 T.B. Cooley and P. Lee, "A series of cases of splenomegaly in children with anemia and peculiar bone changes," *Trans Am Pediatr Soc* 37:29, 1925

30 G.H. Wipple and W.L. Bradford, "Mediterranean disease - thalassemia (erythroblastic anemia of Cooley); associated pigment abnormalities simulating hemochromatosis," *J Pediatr* 9:279-311, 1936.

thalassemia trait. Normally an individual with sickle-cell trait will have both Hb A and Hb S. The usual ratio is not 1:1, as one might expect, but 3:2. This means there is a slight favoring of the production of the normal beta chain over that of the beta chain in Hb S. As a consequence the blood of an AS individual will contain 60% A and 40% S. If, however, an individual with sickle-cell trait also inherits a thalassemia trait, the blood will contain 70-80% Hb S and 20-30% Hb A. Although this person has inherited one gene with the correct genetic code for the beta chain, that gene has some defect that results in the reduced production of normal beta chains.

In 1955 Kunkel and Wallenius[31] noted that Hb $A_2$ is elevated in individuals who carry the thalassemia trait. Since Hb $A_2$ contains two alpha chains and two delta, its production is not influenced by the quantity of beta chains present. If there is a decrease in beta chain production there will be a relative decrease in the quantity of Hb A compared to Hb $A_2$, and the percentage of Hb $A_2$ in the blood will be elevated above the normal range.

Reports also started to appear during the 1950's describing people from Asia with a thalassemia that differed from that seen in Mediterranean regions. In one particular Chinese family there was no elevation of Hb $A_2$, but the investigators discovered a new hemoglobin variant, Hb H, that consisted of four beta chains.

Finally, in 1959 a paper by Ingram and Stretton[32] resolved some of this confusion by dividing thalassemias into two categories: alpha and beta. Each type of thalassemia is caused by reduced production of its corresponding globin chain. While both conditions are seen around the world, beta-thalassemias are most common in the Mediterranean and alpha-thalassemias in Asia.

To understand the basis of the thalassemias on a cellular level it is necessary to look again at the process by which genetic information is transferred and used. The DNA molecule that forms the chromosome carries a sequence of bases (G, C, A and T) that encode the amino acid sequences of proteins. This code is transcribed to an RNA molecule which is then used by the cell to manufacture a protein. The general process is thus:

---

31 H.G. Kunckel and G. Wallenius, "New hemoglobin in adult normal blood," *Science* 122:288, 1955.

32 V. M. Ingram and A.O.W. Stretton, "Genetic basis of the thalassemia disease," *Nature* 184:1903-1909, 1959.

*transcription*              *translation*


DNA →→→→→ RNA →→→→→ protein


The RNA molecule that carries the code from the DNA in the chromosome out to the ribosomes for translation is called the messenger RNA or mRNA.

There are two possible situations that can cause a thalassemia. There can be a <u>deletion</u> of that segment of the DNA molecule that codes for the globin chain, or there can be a <u>mutation</u> somewhere in the DNA code that alters the amount of globin chain produced. In the first condition there can be no production of globin chains because a section of the DNA molecule with the amino acid sequence has been lost. It is gone forever. In the nondeletional case, the globin gene is present, but there has been a mutation or deletion of the DNA surrounding the gene. This mutation alters the <u>rate</u> at which the correct globin is produced. Both these possible situations are found in the different thalassemias.

The information for the manufacture of beta chains is found on chromosome 11. On this same chromosome are the codes for the beta-like globins: the embryonic epsilon ($\in$), the two[†] gamma ($\gamma$) chains used during fetal life, and the delta ($\delta$) chain found in Hb $A_2$. Between the segments that code for the specific chains there are a large number of sequences that code for other proteins or else are just meaningless. (Figure 32.)

The genetics of sickle-cell anemia is explained by the existence of a single mutation at one point on chromosome 11 where the code for the sixth amino acid of the beta globin is located. The result is an amino acid different from the normal; one that gives the hemoglobin molecule some instability in a low oxygen environment.

Studies of individuals with beta-thalassemia generally indicated that the beta globin gene was there, intact, and correct. Instead, the problem appeared to be caused by a deficiency in the output of mRNA molecules. These mRNA deficiencies were due to errors in the code surrounding the beta-globin gene — errors that affected the information needed to manufacture the RNA.

---

† For some reason there are two genes controlling the production of gamma chains. The two chains are not identical but differ by one amino acid at position 136.

## Figure 32. Chromosome 11

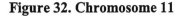

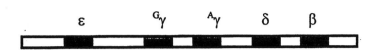

Chromosome 11 contains the DNA codes for the embryonic hemoglobin epsilon ($\epsilon$) chain, two fetal gamma ($\gamma$) chains that differ by only one amino acid, the delta ($\delta$) chain in Hb $A_2$ and the normal beta ($\beta$) chain.

Thus far over 140 specific genetic conditions have been found to cause beta-thalassemia. A few are deletional, but the majority are nondeletional. An example of the latter is a frameshift mutation. When the cell is making mRNA from the DNA template there are certain base sequences that indicate where the code for a protein starts and where it stops. These are known as initiation and termination codons. A change in these codons (like the loss of a base or the addition of an extra one) will confuse the chemistry of the process. The cell cannot tell where to start or where to stop the RNA molecule. The resulting mRNA molecule, if any is even produced, will be too long and will not produce the proper beta chain.

Some mutations yield no beta chains at all; a few result in reduced production of beta chains. This difference helps to explain some of the variability seen in individuals with beta-thalassemia. To distinguish the two forms, the condition where no beta chains are formed is denoted $\beta^0$-thalassemia. If there is production of beta chains in reduced quantities it is $\beta^+$-thalassemia.

The various genetic mutations that cause beta-thalassemia are not evenly distributed around the world. Each ethnic group has its own set of mutations. Those that are seen in Italians and Sicilians are not the same as those found in southeast Asians.

The pattern of inheritance for beta-thalassemia, regardless of the mutation, is basically similar to that for sickle-cell anemia. Each person receives from each parent a chromosome with the information needed to produce beta chains. Thus the normal individual will have two chromosomes directing the synthesis of normal beta chains at a normal rate. If, however, one of the parents donates a chromosome with deletions or mutations that result in a reduced beta chain production, the individual is a carrier of the beta-thalassemia trait. Such a person is heterozygous, i.e., the two genes are not the same. If both parents donate a beta-thalassemia gene, the offspring will be homozygous for the disorder.

People who carry the trait do not suffer any serious adverse health effects. There is only a slight reduction in total beta-chain production. The cell recognizes that one gene is defective and increases output from the other. But there will be, in the end, some slight reduction in the total number of hemoglobin molecules in most of the red cells, and a mild form of anemia may be present in the heterozygote. They generally have no other symptoms to indicate they might be carriers. Laboratory studies will reveal red cells that are slightly smaller in size and lighter in color than normal. Otherwise carriers can easily lead a normal life of normal length and never have any reason to suspect they carry the trait.

As in sickle-cell anemia, the marriage of two people who carry the trait can produce a homozygous child with beta-thalassemia. The homozygous state is a much more serious condition. The severity of the reduction in beta-chain production will depend on the particular deletional or nondeletional mutation inherited. It is not easily recognized at birth because the hemoglobin in the newborn is mostly Hb F, which has no beta chain. However, soon after birth the body switches the production of chains and beta chains are supposed to replace gamma.

The child with beta-thalassemia soon develops severe anemia. The spleen and liver grow progressively larger, giving the child a 'bloated-belly' look. The body, recognizing that it is not receiving adequate supplies of oxygen, will attempt to produce more and more erythrocytes. Bone marrow will expand beyond normal size and distort bones. When this happens in the skull and facial bones, the result is a Mongoloid appearance. In addition, the longer bones have thinner walls and fracture easily. A child with beta-thalassemia will often suffer from ulcers, gallstones and recurring infections. Physical growth and development will be seriously impaired.

Children with beta-thalassemia seldom survive beyond their teenage years. The only treatment found so far that is in any way effective is to transfuse the child with normal blood on a regular basis. However, this treatment creates its own difficulties. The repeated transfusion of blood into a person over a long period can result in the accumulation of excessive quantities of iron in the body. This iron overload can damage the heart, liver, pancreas and other organs. The result can be cardiac failure for those who survive into their twenties unless iron levels are reduced through some type of iron chelation therapy.

About 1,000 people in the United States have homozygous beta-thalassemia. The trait and the disease are found primarily among people whose ancestors come from Mediterranean countries (Italy, Sicily, Spain and Greece) and Africa. There are some areas of the world where a very high percentage of the people carry the trait. In some regions of Italy 20% of the people are carriers. Naturally the number of children with the disease is also very high in these regions. Beta-thalassemia trait is also found to some extent in the Middle East, China, southeast Asia, and India. Worldwide there may be 140,000 people with homozygous beta-thalassemia.

People with ethnic backgrounds in which there is a high frequency of beta-thalassemia may wish to know if they or their spouse carry the trait. This will help them make more informed decisions about family planning, prenatal screening, etc. One of the easiest ways to test for the beta-thalassemia trait is to measure the concentration of Hb $A_2$ in the blood. A normal individual will have 1.5 – 3.0% Hb $A_2$. In carriers of the beta-thalassemia trait there is a slight reduction in beta chain synthesis, and no change in delta chain production. The result is a relative increase in Hb $A_2$ levels to between 3.5 and 10.0%.

Like beta-thalassemia, alpha-thalassemia is a hereditary disorder that results in the reduced production of globin chains, specifically the alpha. However, this disorder is complicated by the fact that there are _four_ genes controlling alpha chain production in a normal individual.

The codes for the alpha and alpha-like globins are located on chromosome 16. On each side of the chromosome (the maternal and the paternal) there are two sites that contain the exact same sequence for alpha chains: $\alpha 1$ and $\alpha 2$. Both sites are functional, but they do not produce equal numbers of globin chains. Expression of the $\alpha 2$ gene is actually three times that for $\alpha 1$. This means that 25% of the alpha chains in a red cell come from the $\alpha 1$ gene and 75% from the $\alpha 2$.

The genetic mutations that cause beta-thalassemia are primarily nondeletional changes that alter the production of mRNA. In contrast, the alpha-thalassemias are due primarily to deletions of large segments of DNA. Somewhere in the past a large section of DNA was lost from chromosome 16, and this lost section included the code for one or both alpha genes.

Over 40 mutations have been identified that cause alpha-thalassemia. A few are nondeletional and affect the production of mRNA from one or both genes. The majority are deletional and include either one or both sites. (Figure 33.)

A person with beta-thalassemia is either homozygous or heterozygous. There are only two possible genetic states. The variability of the disorder comes with the extent of reduction in beta-chain production between the more than 140 mutations. Alpha-thalassemia is further complicated by the existence of two genes on each chromosome producing unequal quantities of alpha chains. In addition, while there can obviously be no chain production in a deletional mutation, the nondeletional mutations can result in the same variability of gene expression as seen in beta-thalassemia.

The normal individual, having four genes, two on each chromosome, is described as $\alpha\alpha/\alpha\alpha$. If a gene is missing or inactivated it is replaced with a "-". Thus alpha-thalassemia can be the result of one ($-\alpha/\alpha\alpha$), two ($-\alpha/-\alpha$ or $--/\alpha\alpha$), three ($--/-\alpha$) or four ($--/--$) gene deletions. Each condition will be covered in more detail.

The simplest and least harmful alpha-thalassemia is $-\alpha/\alpha\alpha$. Only one of the three genes is missing, and there is very little decrease in total globin chain production. This condition, heterozygous alpha-thalassemia-2, is so mild that it is often called the silent carrier. Most people do not even know they carry this trait. The worst consequence of inheriting this gene pattern is a very mild anemia. Heterozygous alpha-thalassemia-2 is extremely common in some regions of the world. It is especially high in black Africans. Studies indicated that 30% of Afro-Americans are carriers of this trait.

**Figure 33. Chromosome 16**

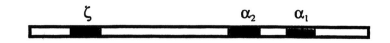

Chromosome 16 contains the DNA codes for the embryonic zeta ($\dot{\omega}$) chain and the two alpha chains ($\alpha_1$ and $\alpha_2$).

The homozygous form of alpha-thalassemia-2 (-α/-α) with its two missing genes is only slightly more serious. Once again the worst result is a mild anemia.

It is also possible to have two missing alpha genes on the same chromosome (- -/αα). This condition is the heterozygous form of alpha-thalassemia-1. It is very important to see the genetic difference between -α/-α and --/αα. The two missing genes in homozygous alpha-thalassemia-2 (-α/-α) are on separate chromosomes. That individual cannot donate a chromosome with both genes missing. The heterozygous alpha-thalassemia-1, on the other hand, has one normal chromosome (αα) and one with no alpha genes (--). Either chromosome can be donated to an offspring.

If two people who are heterozygous for alpha-thalassemia-1 have children, there is a 25% probability that any one of their offspring will inherit both chromosomes with no alpha genes. This homozygous state of alpha-thalassemia-1 (--/--) has no genes for the production of alpha chains. This is fatal because the body cannot survive without alpha chains.

Alpha-thalassemia-1 is found with high frequency in southeast Asia. There is very little in the United States except in areas where there are people whose ancestors came from southeast Asia. In Thailand alone there are over 15,000 cases a year of babies born with homozygous alpha-thalassemia-1. These babies are usually stillborn or die shortly after birth. The condition is known as hydrops fetalis.

Finally, it is also possible to have an alpha-thalassemia with three genes deleted. This can occur when someone inherits both an alpha-thalassemia-1 (- -) and an alpha-thalassemia-2 (-α) gene. The result (- -/-α) leaves only one functioning alpha gene, and there is significant reduction in alpha chain production. The red cell produces an excess of beta chains. Under these conditions the beta chains will start to combine with each other to form an unstable hemoglobin molecule. This is the hemoglobin H (β$_4$) mentioned earlier that was found in the Chinese family with alpha-thalassemia. Because of its presence the disorder has been named hemoglobin H disease even though the H is merely a by-product of the condition.

Unfortunately the Hb H does not take the place of normal hemoglobin. It can carry oxygen to some extent, but it is an unstable molecule and tends to precipitate inside the red cell. Someone with Hb H disease tends to have rather serious anemia. It is the only alpha-thalassemia condition that can, or needs to be, treated.

If it is possible for a $\beta_4$ hemoglobin to form, can there also be a $\gamma_4$? The gamma chain is like beta in length and function, so it would seem that when the gamma gene is operating in a fetus with alpha-thalassemia there will be excess gamma chains produced. Investigators at St. Bartholomew's Hospital in London reported in 1958 that they had found a new hemoglobin variant in a 9-month old baby. This new variant contained four gamma chains and was named hemoglobin Bart's after the hospital where it was first identified.

In a normal fetus there is often a slight overproduction of gamma chains, and there will be 0-1% Hb Bart's at birth. If heterozygous alpha-thalassemia-2 is present ($\alpha\alpha/-\alpha$), the Bart's concentration will be between 1 and 3%. Two deletions (i.e., either $-\alpha/-\alpha$ or $-/\alpha\alpha$) will result in 3-9% Hb Bart's. The three deletion condition that will become Hb H disease in the adult is revealed by seeing 25% Hb Bart's in the newborn. Finally, in hydrops fetalis (homozygous alpha-thalassemia-1), where there is no alpha-chain production, Hb Bart's will be the major hemoglobin and will form 80% or more of the total. Unfortunately the Hb Bart's is not able to transport sufficient oxygen to the cells and cannot replace Hb A. The other hemoglobins in a hydrops fetalis baby will be embryonic types that have not been completely switched off. They also cannot satisfy the newborn's need for oxygen.

# Chapter 8

# THE MAJOR GENETIC VARIANTS

The thalassemias discussed in the previous chapter are all the result of an inherited defect in the rate of production of normal globin chains. A different type of disorder can occur when the genetic code does not carry the correct information for the proper sequence of amino acids in one of the globin chains. The result is the production of an abnormal chain and, consequently, an abnormal hemoglobin variant. Normal hemoglobin components F and $A_2$ are produced by the body under the control of normal genetic codes. Abnormal hemoglobin variants are the result of abnormal codes.

The pattern of inheritance for a hemoglobin variant is generally similar to that already described for beta-thalassemia and sickle-cell anemia. Each individual has two genetic patterns to specify the amino acid sequence in each globin chain for the adult hemoglobin: one set of four genes for the alpha chain and one set of two genes for the beta chain. Each parent has contributed half of each set.

If an individual inherits one abnormal gene (or set of genes) and one normal gene, that person is a carrier of the trait. There is a 50% chance that the trait will be passed on to each child. As before, those who only carry the trait are called heterozygous. On the other hand, an individual who possesses two genes of the same type, whether they are normal or abnormal, will be homozygous. If the two genes both result in one specific globin chain with an abnormality, the person will be homozygous for that variant. This individual will certainly pass the trait on to any children.

So far there have been over 700 hemoglobin chain variants discovered. Some are widespread and occur in millions of people in the world. Others have been found in only a few related families. The consequences of having an hemoglobin variant can range from very seriously affecting the individual's health, as in sickle-cell anemia, to having no noticeable influence at all.

These abnormal hemoglobins arise because of a mutation in the genetic code. Exactly how these mutations occur is not known. But they can occur — some more readily than others — and once they do occur they can be passed on to succeeding generations unless the mutation is so serious that the individual does not survive to adulthood.

Hemoglobin variants were first named by using letters. The first variant found to differ from normal adult hemoglobin was the fetal hemoglobin of a newborn. To distinguish between the two the adult's was designated Hb A while the fetus' was Hb F. Pauling and his associates called the hemoglobin responsible for sickle-cell anemia hemoglobin S. This use of single letters to indicate a hemoglobin variant continued until there were obviously going to be more variants than letters in the alphabet. There was no agreed upon method, but generally the discoverers of new variants began to use the names of cities or regions where the variant was discovered. Sometimes the name was used by itself, as in Hb Malmö, and other times it was added to a letter, as in Hb G-Philadelphia.

Soon, because of independent discoveries by several investigators, several names were being used to describe what was later found to be the same variant. The terms J-Baltimore, J- Trinidad, J-Ireland, J-New Haven, and J-Georgia all apply to the exact same variant. Each time it was given a new name by someone who thought they had discovered a new variant.

Now scientists generally attach to a common name (like J-Baltimore) an exact description of the amino acid substitution that has created the variant. In the case of J-Baltimore the 16th amino acid of the beta chain, which should be glycine (gly), has been replaced by aspartic acid (asp). This is indicated as $\beta16$ gly $\rightarrow$ asp. In modern medical literature the variant is thus usually described by using both the common name and the substitution, i.e., Hb J-Baltimore ($\beta16$ gly $\rightarrow$ asp). With this system there is no confusion as to exactly which variant is being discussed.

The rest of this chapter will review some of the major hemoglobin variants in the world. The primary concern will be the effect the presence of the abnormal hemoglobin has on the health of the individual in both the homozygous and heterozygous cases. While some typical symptoms will be mentioned in connection with each variant, it is important to remember that these are only generalities. There are many other factors that can lessen or increase the severity of a hemoglobin variant. Any person who has or suspects they have inherited a hemoglobin variant should seek professional medical help for thorough testing and counseling.

Detection and identification of the major hemoglobin variants is fairly easy. Most hospital laboratories have the ability to detect and identify the common variants. There are several specialized labs in the country that routinely do the more complicated tests that produce the exact amino acid sequence needed to precisely identify a variant.

# HEMOGLOBIN S ($\beta$6 GLU $\rightarrow$ VAL)

Hb S is responsible for the most widely known and most common hemoglobinopathy in the United States — sickle-cell anemia. Approximately 1 out of every 10 American Blacks are carriers (i.e., they are heterozygous) for Hb S. This gene is part of their African heritage. In some areas of Africa today as many as 40% of the population are carriers of the sickle-cell anemia trait.

Estimates indicate that about 30 million people in the world carry the gene for Hb S. Although it is most often found in peoples of African descent, it also appears in Italians, Turks, Greeks, Arabs, and Asian Indians.

The basic sickling character of red cells with Hb S was already discussed in Chapter 1. Individuals with sickle-cell trait usually encounter no health problems. There may be some sickled cells in the blood and some slight symptoms of anemia, but the individual generally leads a normal life of normal length. There has been some concern that in very stressful situations or during times of low oxygen availability to the cells, there can be a significant amount of sickling even in someone who only is a carrier. However, this has never really been shown to be the case.

However, if two people who are carriers marry and have children, the chances are 25% that each child will inherit the gene from both parents, be homozygous for Hb S, and have sickle-cell anemia. This condition is much more serious than just having the trait. Approximately 70,000 people in the United States have sickle-cell anemia.

People with sickle-cell anemia produce no hemoglobin A. Their red cells contain mostly Hb S along with some Hb F and a small amount of Hb $A_2$. The Hb S differs from normal Hb A in that the sixth amino acid in the beta chain is valine rather than glutamic acid. This seems like such a minor difference, yet this one substitution has a big impact on the health of the individual. How does this happen?

Without delving into the complexities of chemical bonds, three-dimensional structure of hemoglobin, and crystal formation, the easiest approach to a basic understanding of what this one alteration means to Hb S can be found in the following analogy[†]:

Picture Hb A in its oxygenated form, the T state, as a collection of four squares – each square representing one of the globin chains. In the deoxy, or R, state, the molecule changes shape slightly and creates a small depression in each of the alpha chains. Oxy-Hb S is like A except that the valine creates a small "sticky patch" on each beta chain. While the hemoglobin is oxygenated, the sticky patch has nothing to adhere to. However, the deoxy S has the same depressions on the alpha chain that A does, and the sticky patches on the beta chains fit them very nicely. Thus, in a low oxygen environment the Hb S molecules can link together to form long, fiber-like crystals. These crystals grow very long and associate with each other in bundles. The Hb S crystalizes into long needles that distort the red cell membrane and give it a sickle-like shape. (See Figure 34.)

These sickled cells will not flow through the blood vessels as easily as normal red cells. They tend to clog small capillaries and block the flow of blood. This can produce swelling and pain in the joints and often causes headaches and dizziness. People with sickle-cell anemia also have problems fighting infections. They have to be extra careful to avoid catching colds, flu, etc.

---

† See *Molecular Design of Life*, Lubert Stryer, W.H. Freeman, New York, 1988, pp 166-167.

## Figure 34. The Formation of Hb S Crystals

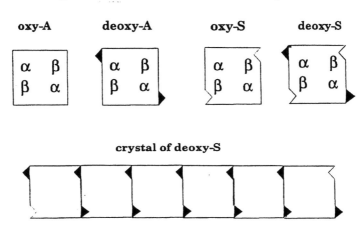

crystal of deoxy-S

Although there is no known cure for sickle-cell anemia, there are many things that can be done to lessen its severity. Intelligent care of the disease will reduce suffering and decrease mortality. Analgesics can be used to reduce pain. Children can be vaccinated and antibiotics can be used to help combat infections, especially in the early years. In more serious sickling conditions physicians may transfuse normal blood into the patient at regular intervals. With good nutrition, plenty of liquids, and avoidance of extremes of both hot and cold weather, a person with sickle-cell anemia may reduce the frequency and severity of attacks. High levels of physical activity will deplete oxygen in the blood, and reduced levels of oxygen increase the potential for sickling. Some individuals may have to limit their physical activities and participation in sports to control their condition.

The patients themselves monitor their activities and their habits and by their own efforts help reduce the affects of their disorder. Sickle-cell anemia does not affect every individual the same way. Some people live to old age with only a few painful bouts of sickling crises. Others will suffer greatly for years before an early death.

People with sickle-cell anemia have the usual range of intelligence. They should be encouraged to live up to their intellectual potential and to engage in a level of physical activity (at work and at play) that is consistent with the severity of their disease. Living with sickle-cell anemia can be a serious burden, but it can often be a manageable situation. The child, the adolescent, and the adult with homozygous Hb S must realize that they are different from those around them and take extra precautions to protect their health.

Even though all the research on hemoglobin has not produced a cure for sickle-cell anemia, we do seem to be close to developing methods for masking the disorder by modifying the body's chemistry to compensate for the genetic mutation.

It has already been noted that in 1948 Janet Watson suggested that hemoglobin might be the cause of sickle-cell anemia. She had observed that newborns, with high levels of Hb F, had fewer sickled cells than adults even though both had sickle-cell anemia. She correctly suggested that Hb F inhibits the sickling of cells.

After birth the production of Hb F stops and the gene for producing Hb A (or Hb S) is turned on. However, the cells still possess the genes that contain the information needed to make Hb F. In fact, some people do not completely shut down the production of Hb F. Sickle-cell anemia has been found to be a very mild disorder in some areas of Saudi Arabia. It appears that these people have inherited an ability to increase Hb F production as adults when they have inherited sickle-cell anemia. In this region many adults with sickle-cell anemia will have 10-25% Hb F in their blood. These high levels of Hb F prevent the cells from sickling.

From this observation it would follow that if we could turn on the Hb F gene we could "cure" sickle-cell anemia. Studies are underway to evaluate several methods for increasing levels of Hb F in individuals with sickle-cell anemia. If a method could be found that would increase Hb F levels to above 20% in people with sickle-cell anemia, the severity of the disease would be significantly decreased. It would not, of course, actually cure the disease. It would only eliminate the worst symptoms of the condition.

Because there has been so much confusion about sickle-cell anemia, many do not understand the distinction between those who are only carriers of the trait (i.e., AS) and those who have the disorder (i.e., who are SS). Those who have the trait should not be made to suffer any added insurance costs, employment discrimination, or any feelings of guilt. It has simply happened, by chance, that it is their lot to carry an abnormal gene that will have little, if any, influence on their own health.

However, carriers can pass this trait on to their children. It is important for people to know if they are carriers. If a carrier plans to have children with another carrier, it is only fair that they should be aware of the situation and the possibilities.

# HB C ($\beta$6 GLU → LYS)

Soon after Hb S was discovered and identified, another hemoglobin with an amino acid substitution in the sixth position of the beta chain was found. It was called Hb C. In this case, the glutamic acid normally found at beta 6 is replaced by lysine. Hb C is found in 2-3% of American Blacks. For some unexplained reason it is more common in women than in men at a ratio of 3:1.

With the Hb C trait (AC) people experience no clinical symptoms. The heterozygous condition is completely benign. About one in 6,000 Blacks has Hb C disease (CC). They may experience a moderate degree of anemia and mild forms of the symptoms of sickle-cell anemia. In some regions of Africa the frequency of Hb C trait is 20%. It can also be found in Italians, Greeks, Turks and Arabs.

# HB E ($\beta$26 GLU → LYS)

Hemoglobin E is the third most frequently seen hemoglobin variant in the United States, but world-wide it may be more common than Hb S. Approximately 30 million people are thought to have Hb E disease (EE) or trait (AE). Hb E occurs with greatest frequency in southeast Asia and appears to be limited to people whose ancestors came from that region.

Hb E trait is very innocuous and produces few, if any, symptoms. Homozygous Hb E is also not very serious. The individual with Hb E disease (EE) may show some symptoms of slight anemia because the E beta chains are not synthesized as fast as the beta A chains. Hence, there is a slight decrease in the total hemoglobin in the blood.

# HB D (β121 GLU → GLN)

Hemoglobin D is often called Hb D-Los Angeles (where it was first discovered) and Hb D-Punjab (where it is most common). In the Punjab region of India and Pakistan approximately 3% of the people are carriers of the trait. It is also found in the British Isles — partly as a result of the intermarriage between British and Indians during the British occupation of the area, but also as a result of immigration to the United Kingdom. In North America the trait occurs in fewer than 1 out of 5,000 people.

Hb D trait has no clinical manifestations. The homozygous form is rare and fairly mild.

# HB G-PHILADELPHIA (α68 ASN → LYS)

All the hemoglobin variants mentioned thus far have been the result of amino acid substitutions in the beta chain. Hb G-Philadelphia is the most common variant involving alpha chains. It is the only alpha chain variant seen with any real frequency in the U.S. Hb G-Philadelphia appears to be limited to American and African Blacks and has not been seen in other ethnic groups. It is found in approximately 1 in 5,000 black Americans. Both the trait and the homozygous form are benign and show no adverse clinical symptoms.

The existence of four alpha globin genes complicates the amount of Hb G-Philadelphia found in heterozygotes. It was noted in the previous chapter that each person normally inherits two alpha genes from each parent and is thus described as αα/αα. If the individual has an alpha-thalassemia, a "-" indicates a missing gene. Thus, α-/αα is heterozygous alpha-thalassemia-2, --/αα is heterozygous alpha-thalassemia-1, α-/α- is homozygous alpha-thalassemia-2, --/-- is homozygous alpha-thalassemia-1 (hydrops fetalis), and α-/-- is Hemoglobin H disease. The G-Philadelphia trait appears to be frequently associated with an alpha-thalassemia: there is a gene with a coding error ($\alpha^G$) and a missing alpha gene on the chromosome. Such an individual, if heterozygous, would be -$\alpha^G$/αα. Since the alpha-thalassemia-2 gene is common among black Americans, the combination -$\alpha^G$/-α is often found. These people will have 40% Hb G-Philadelphia and 60% Hb A. This is similar to sickle cell trait, $\beta^S$/β, where 40% Hb S and 60% Hb A are typical.

When a person has the $-\alpha^G/$ chromosome matched with a normal chromosome, they will be $-\alpha^G/\alpha\alpha$ and usually produce 30% G-Philadelphia. The two normal genes on the one chromosome outproduce the single variant gene. Finally, when the variant gene is not accompanied by a missing alpha gene (i.e., $\alpha\alpha^G/\alpha\alpha$), there is only 20% G-Philadelphia.

These complications are a matter of scientific interest and help us better understand the genetics of hemoglobin production. They have no influence on the health of those who carry the Hb G-Philadelphia trait.

## HB KÖLN ($\beta$98 VAL → MET)

In northern Europe one of the most common hemoglobin variants is Hb Köln. It appears to be associated with people of German, Dutch or English ancestry and has not been found in any other ethnic groups. Hb Köln trait can produce mild anemia but, in general, does not cause any real disabilities.

## HB M DISORDERS

Although they are not particularly common, Hb M disorders are interesting because of their effect on the individual, even in the heterozygous state. There are over 20 Hb M variants, and they all involve an amino acid substitution that permits the iron to hold on more tightly to the oxygen. Thus, two of the heme-globin units will not give up oxygen, or will yield it with reluctance. The other two chains are normal and do transport oxygen, but the heme-heme interactions are restricted.

In 1948 Hörlein and Weber[33] reported on a family that had several people with a bluish tint to their skin. The blue coloration was especially noticeable around the lips and fingers. These symptoms are similar to those seen in someone poisoned by cyanide and are the result of reduced delivery of oxygen to the tissues. The general term for this condition is *cyanosis*. The investigators found that the hemoglobin in the blood of the affected

---

33 H. Hörlein and G. Weber, "Über chronische familiäre Methämoglobinämie und eine neue Modifikation des Methämoblobins. *Dtsch Med Wochenschr* 73:476, 1948

individuals had some unusual properties, including a dark, or brownish, color. They attributed the condition to a problem with the hemoglobin molecule. This is the first recorded description of a disorder caused by a hemoglobin variant as it preceded the work by Pauling and his associates by a year. It was later discovered that the family had Hb M-Saskatoon (β63 his → tyr).

A similar inherited condition with cyanosis had been observed in Japan since the nineteenth century. It was known as "Kochikuro" (black mouth) or "Chikuro" (black blood). It was found in the 1950s to be caused by a Hb M with an amino acid substitution (his → tyr) at α87 and named M-Iwate after the region in which the carriers lived[34].

Some Hb M variants involve amino acid substitutions on the alpha chain, others on the beta. Only heterozygous Hb M individuals have been found. It is assumed that the homozygous form is not compatible with life. Cyanosis (reduced oxygen delivery) is the only clinical manifestation, and no other disabilities have been noted.

## HB CONSTANT SPRINGS

While the DNA molecules in the chromosomes contain all the codes for the proteins manufactured by the body, they also have millions of bases that do not seem to have any use. They have no apparent function, at least in this stage of human evolution, except to fill in the spaces between the various genes. The cells have biochemical mechanisms to find and copy those sections of DNA that they need. The rest are ignored.

To mark where a code for a protein starts and stops there are special initiation and termination codons. (A codon is a set of three bases.) For example, at the end of the α2 globin gene are the following codons: -ATG-GCA-ATT. The ATG codes for the amino acid tyrosine, the GCA is arginine, and the ATT is a termination codon. The cell reads the DNA and knows that the last two amino acids in the globin chain are tyrosine and arginine.

If, however, there is a mutation and ATT becomes GTT, the cell reads the GTT as the code for glutamic acid and continues to copy the code. More codons are added to the mRNA being produced until a termination codon is

---

34 *Hemoglobin: Molecular, Genetic and Clinical Aspects*, H. Franklin Bunn and Bernard G. Forget, W. B. Saunders Company, Philadelphia, 1986.

reached on the DNA molecule. This is what happens in an individual with Hb Constant Spring. There has been a mutation at the termination codon for the α2 gene and the resulting protein chain contains 31 extra amino acids.

Although the hemoglobin molecule produced with the extended alpha chain is stable, the carriers of Hb Constant Spring usually have only 1-2% of the variant in their blood. It appears that the mRNA formed as a result of the mutation is not stable. Few of the mutant mRNA molecules survive to be translated into proteins in the cytoplasm.

Hb Constant Spring is found in relatively high frequency in southeast Asia and, by itself, presents no health problem. However, it is often seen in conjunction with an alpha-thalassemia, and its presence is essentially the same as if a gene were missing. Thus, someone with Hb Constant Spring trait and alpha-thalassemia-1 trait (i.e., $\alpha^{CS}\alpha$/--) has only one fully functioning alpha gene and will have the symptoms of someone with Hb H disease ($\alpha$-/--).

## HB LEPORE

This is the last type of mutation to be covered in this basic introduction to hemoglobin variants. All the hemoglobin variants mentioned thus far have been the result of a mutation in the sequence of bases on the DNA molecules. The mutation either alters the amino acid for which the DNA molecule codes or eliminates a stop codon and results in an extended chain. The mutation that produces Hb Lepore is different. This variant has a globin chain that starts as a delta and finishes as a beta – the two codes have been fused together as a result of a mutation that occurs during the production of the reproductive cells (i.e., the sperm and the egg).

The majority of the cells in the body contain two sets of chromosomes unless, like the mature red cells, they have no nucleus at all. One set comes from each parent. Each chromosome is attached to its corresponding match from the other parent. Chromosome 11 has both the maternal and the paternal versions lying side by side in the nucleus. However, when reproductive cells are formed by the process of meiosis, they must have only one set of chromosomes. That way, when the reproductive cells combine the offspring will have only one set from each parent.

During meiosis the chromosomes in the nucleus line up with the partners and prepare to split. (See Figure 35.) Just before that occurs the cell "shuffles" the genes. The DNA molecules are cut into pieces which are the randomly reassembled. The original maternal chromosome now contains some of the paternal genes, and visa versa. Each chromosome in the reproductive cells is not just a copy of the chromosome inherited from one of the parents. It contains genes from both. This technique of reshuffling the genes is nature's way of ensuring and promoting genetic diversity.

**Figure 35. Chromosome 11 Before Normal Meiosis**

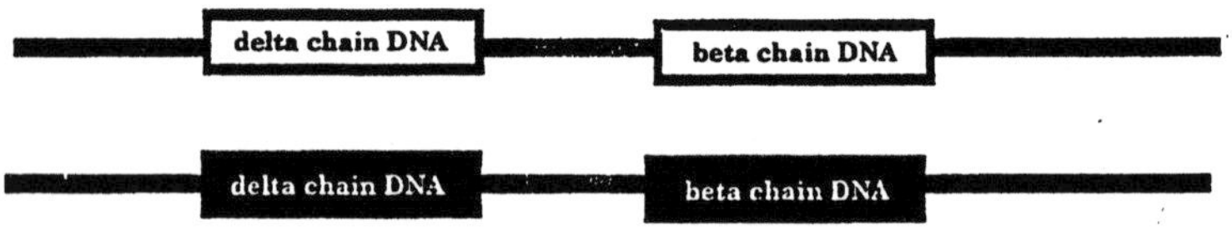

When the chromosomes are about ready to undergo the reshuffling, they line up with corresponding genes across from each other. In particular, on chromosome 11 the delta ($\delta$) and beta ($\beta$) globin genes are lined up as in Figure 35. Because these genes are so similar in their base sequences, it is possible, although very rare, for there to be a misalignment. In such a situation the delta on one chromosome finds itself opposite the beta on the other. During the shuffling of the genes, there is an a fusion of the two. One chromosome ends up with only one gene producing a globin that starts as a $\delta$ chain and finishes as a $\beta$. The other chromosome has extra genetic material. It contains a normal $\beta$, and normal $\delta$, and a fused $\beta\delta$ gene. (Figure 36.)

The $\delta\beta$ fusion product is Hb Lepore. There have actually been three different Hb Lepores discovered. They differ from each other as to the actual place on the chain where the fusion occurs. Someone with Hb Lepore will produce 10-15% of the variant, and the trait condition is similar to the beta-thalassemia trait. It has little, if any, effect on the health of the carrier.

The other chromosome is the anti-Lepore. That individual has a normal beta chain and can produce normal hemoglobin. They may have a small amount of a hemoglobin variant with a $\beta\delta$ fusion, but it is of no consequence to their health.

**Figure 36. Formation of Hb Lepore and Anti-Lepore**

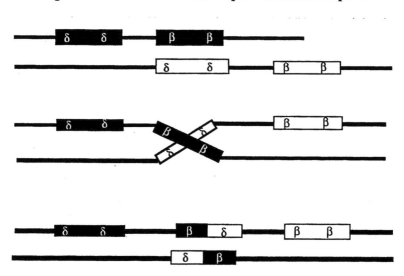

## OTHER HEMOGLOBIN VARIANTS AND COMBINATIONS

While it is true that hundreds of hemoglobin variants have been omitted from this discussion, most of them are very rare and the symptoms are relatively mild. However, it should be mentioned that individuals can be heterozygous for two different hemoglobin variants or for both a hemoglobin variant and a thalassemia. For example, if an AS individual marries an AC, the following combinations are possible in their children: AA, AS, AC, SC. In the U.S. the most frequently seen combinations are those seen with Hb S, particularly SC, SG-Philadelphia and S-beta-thalassemia. In Southeast Asia Hb E trait and EE disease are frequently found in individuals who have also inherited alpha- or beta-thalassemia.

## GEOGRAPHICAL DISTRIBUTION

Hemoglobin variants and thalassemias are found throughout the world[35]. The frequency of each condition varies with the ethnic and racial mix of the people in that region. While Africa, India, southeast Asia, and China have particularly large numbers of variants, there is no nation or race that is without its own set of variants. However, the major variants that do affect the health of individuals have been covered. Hemoglobins S and E in their homozygous state and when associated with other variants and with thalassemias constitute the major problems. Most of the other variants are found only as heterozygotes or have very little affect on health even in the homozygous form.

---

35 *Human Variants in Human Populations,* Vols I and II, William Winter (ed), CRC Press, Inc., Boca Raton, FL, 1986.

# Chapter 9

# DIABETES AND HEMOGLOBIN

Each individual inherits the ability to produce several different hemoglobin variants during life. The genetic code carries information as to what sequence of amino acids will be used to form the globin chains. The code also determines the rate at which hemoglobin is synthesized and manipulates the switching mechanism that stops the production of one variant and starts that of another. During early embryonic life the human fetus produces a series of different hemoglobins as needed. Manufacture of the final fetal hemoglobin (Hb F) is turned off at birth when the body switches to the production of adult hemoglobin.

The previous chapters have discussed the genetic factors that control hemoglobin production and determine the variants produced. If there are any inherited defects, abnormal conditions may result. In thalassemia disorders, normal hemoglobin is produced at a reduced rate. On the other hand, those who inherit a hemoglobin variant manufacture globin chains with abnormal amino acid sequences. How this condition affects their health depends on the nature of the amino acid substitution and whether they are homozygous or heterozygous for the variant.

The term 'hemoglobinopathy' refers to genetic disorders related to the production of hemoglobin and covers both thalassemias and hemoglobin variants.

Once genes with errors in the genetic code have been inherited, there is nothing as yet that medical science can do to prevent the formation of abnormal hemoglobins or alter the rate of synthesis. It may be possible in the future to switch off one gene and activate another, but there is no known way to do this now. Physicians have to concentrate on treating the symptoms of hemoglobinopathies; they cannot yet cure these disorders.

There are also a number of hemoglobin variants that have been found to be produced in the body after the hemoglobin molecule has been synthesized. Since these variants are created after the genetic code has been translated from the DNA molecule, they are called post-translational modifications.

The post-translational variants that have been discovered appear to be products of reactions in the red cell between hemoglobin and other molecules that circulate in the blood. They most often consist of normal hemoglobins (i.e., the normal hemoglobin produced by that particular person) with something attached to it. In some cases this reaction product is irreversible, and the final product is stable. The post-translational variant accumulates in the red cell until the red cell is destroyed. In a few cases the post-translational variant appears to be formed temporarily, and the reaction can be reversed.

These post-translational variants have been investigated only within the last twenty years. Very little is known about most of them. They generally exist in relatively small concentrations and have no effect on the health of the individual. However, they may be valuable for their diagnostic use. Measurement of the concentrations of certain post-translational hemoglobin modifications may be useful in assessing the health of the individual.

One particular group of post-translational variants has received considerable attention. Its most accurate name is glycohemoglobin - usually abbreviated GHb. It is also frequently called glycosylated or glycated hemoglobin.

GHb is formed by the reaction between glucose, a sugar that circulates freely in the blood, and hemoglobin[36]. There are several places along the globin chain where glucose can form a permanent attachment to the hemoglobin molecule. Hence, GHb really includes a group of molecules with different structures, depending on where the glucose is attached, but with the same formula and all created by the same type of reaction.

When a red cell is first formed and placed in the circulating blood stream, it will have all new hemoglobin molecules and no GHb. During its life the red cell will travel through blood containing glucose molecules. These glucose molecules can pass freely through the membrane surrounding the red cell, and

---

36 E. C. Abraham, *Glycosylated Hemoglobins*. New York: Marcel Dekker, Inc., 1985.

the concentration of glucose in the cell will be the same as that in the blood stream outside the cell.

Throughout the 120-days of the red cell's life the glucose will slowly but steadily react with hemoglobin molecules until approximately 14% of the hemoglobin has a glucose attached to it. If we take a random sample of blood and measure the level of GHb, it will be about 7% in a normal adult. Any particular red cell will have a GHb value between 0 and 14%. Since the red cells are randomly mixed in the blood, the average GHb will be about 7%.

If the red cells are exposed to abnormally high concentrations of glucose, this will be reflected in higher GHb levels. For this reason the GHb test has become an important tool for monitoring the therapy of diabetics and for measuring the ability of the body to regulate carbohydrate metabolism.

To appreciate the significance of the GHb assay it is necessary to understand the nature of diabetes and its complications.

Diabetes is a disorder that is known to affect between six and seven million people in the United States. It was recognized by physicians as early as 1500 B.C., but there was no treatment and little understanding of diabetes until the twentieth century. Typical symptoms of diabetes are excessive thirst, frequent urination, and sugar in the urine. Without treatment diabetics lose weight, regardless of how much they eat, and the levels of glucose in the blood rise to dangerous levels. In extreme cases the untreated diabetic might pass into a coma and die.

Diabetes is essentially a disorder in the body's regulation of carbohydrate metabolism. When carbohydrates (i.e., starches and complex sugars) are digested they are broken down into a simple sugar — glucose.. The blood carries the glucose out to the cells and tissues of the body where it is further metabolized to produce water, carbon dioxide, and the energy needed for other cellular processes. When the cells have all the glucose they need, the excess is stored in the liver.

In order to help regulate the levels of glucose in the blood, the pancreas, a small gland near the stomach, produces the hormone insulin. The insulin molecule is like a key that attaches itself to special insulin receptors on the cell membrane and "unlocks" a door to let glucose in. If no insulin is present, glucose concentrations will increase in the blood, but the sugar cannot get into the cells to provide the energy needed.

Normally the pancreas senses a rise in blood glucose levels (e.g., after a meal) and secretes insulin to promote storage of glucose in the liver or entry

of glucose into the cells.  As the blood glucose concentration drops, the output
and concentration of insulin in the blood declines.  People with diabetes are
generally unable to produce insulin fast enough or in sufficient quantities to
keep blood glucose levels normal.  This elevation of glucose concentrations in
the blood can cause both immediate and long-term health problems.

Diabetes is generally broken down into two categories.  Type I diabetics
are insulin-dependent and must rely totally on an external supply of insulin to
regulate their blood glucose.  About one million U.S. diabetics are Type I.
They must take daily injections of insulin to replace that normally produced
by the pancreas.  The Type II diabetic, on the other hand, is not insulin
dependent.  Some may take an oral medication that causes their pancreas to
produce more insulin or else allows the body to make more efficient use of the
insulin it already produces.   Other Type II diabetics can manage their
condition by carefully watching their diet and controlling the rate and
quantities of foods consumed.

Because the diabetic's natural, automatic blood glucose regulatory
mechanism is not working properly, the individual has to consciously do the
regulating.  Physicians evaluate the extent of the disorder and the life style of
the individual to prescribe a regimen that includes medication (if needed),
dietary guidelines, and exercise.  These three factors, if properly balanced,
will help the diabetic achieve blood glucose control as close to normal as
possible.

## Figure 37. Daily Blood Glucose Changes

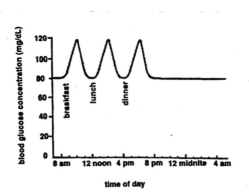

The concentration of glucose in the blood is usually expressed as milligrams (mg) of the sugar per 100 milliliters (mL) of blood. Since 100 mL equals 1 deciliter (dL), the unit is more often expressed as mg/dL. The body tries to keep the level of glucose in the blood between 60 and 100 mg/dL.

Measuring the degree of blood glucose control achieved by a diabetic has always been difficult. One method is to test for sugar (i.e., glucose) in the urine. Many diabetics have used this test at home to check themselves, but it is not a very sensitive assay. Glucose levels in the blood must be twice normal, around 180 mg/dL, before the sugar starts to spill over from the blood into the urine. The major test used for years by physicians has been the blood glucose test. This test measures the amount of glucose in the blood at one particular instant in time. It reflects the degree of immediate blood glucose control.

Unfortunately, blood glucose levels fluctuate from minute to minute, even in a normal individual. For example, the typical non-diabetic person might have a blood glucose concentration of 70 mg/dL on first waking in the morning. After breakfast the value would increase slowly to around 90 or 100. It would then drop down until a new supply of carbohydrates at lunch (or morning coffee break) raises it again. This cycle continues throughout the day. During the night the value drops once again to a low point. (Figure 37.)

Normal blood glucose levels vary during the day between 60 and 100 mg/dL. A diabetic's value may vary from as low as 30 or 40 (usually indicating they have taken too much insulin) to highs of 500 or 600. The level of glucose in the blood for anyone will depend on their medication, exercise, and what they have eaten in the last few hours. It is not a good way to measure how well the diabetic is doing overall.

Unfortunately, physicians in the past really had no choice but to test blood glucose levels when a diabetic came to the office for a visit and base their judgments on the results of this test plus information from the patient concerning their general state of health and the results of any urine sugar tests performed at home by the diabetic. Recently small instruments have been made available that permit diabetics to test their own blood glucose levels at home every day, or even several times during the day, to help them maintain better control. The immediate need in treating diabetes is, of course, to keep blood glucose levels below the danger point. If the concentration of glucose in the blood remains high, it means the cells are starving in the midst of plenty. They cannot obtain the glucose needed for energy. The body becomes tired and lacks the energy to work. Extremely high levels of glucose in the blood result in some chemical by-products that accumulate in the blood and may produce a coma.

After years of experience treating diabetes with insulin, it was noted that some diabetics developed medical complications that seem unrelated to blood glucose levels. Most of the complications related to vascular problems, i.e., they concerned the blood vessels. The *microvascular* problems occurred in the small blood vessels in the eyes, the kidneys, and the nerves. Many diabetics developed problems with their vision, and diabetes became the leading cause of blindness in the United States. Other complications that could develop after years of diabetes included kidney failures and multiple neurological symptoms (pain, burning sensations, and numbness in various parts of the body.) There were, in addition, health problems related to the larger blood vessels that often resulted in reduced blood flow. These *macrovascular* problems could contribute to angina, heart attacks, strokes, and reduced ability to fight infections, especially in the legs. However, not all diabetics would automatically encounter these vascular problems. Some have these complications after years of diabetes; others do not. The difference seemed to be generally correlated to the treating physician's estimate of the general degree of blood glucose control maintained by the diabetic. Those in good control seemed to have fewer long-term complications than those who, for whatever reason, could not keep their blood glucose near normal ranges.

It became apparent that there was a need for a yardstick to monitor and measure long-term blood glucose control in diabetes. Good health management indicated that there is more to diabetes care than just keeping the diabetic alive and glucose levels inside safe ranges. The best treatment would keep the diabetic's blood glucose levels as close to normal as possible. A test was needed to measure degree of blood glucose control over a long period, but nothing was available until the GHb test was invented.

Since GHb is formed by the reaction between hemoglobin and glucose, an increase in the concentration of glucose will result in the formation of more glycohemoglobin. Once this GHb is formed, it will not disappear until the red cell in which it is located is destroyed. Hence, the amount of GHb in a single red cell accurately reflects the amount of glucose that red cell has been exposed to from the beginning of its life in the blood stream. A sample of blood taken at random will contain red cells of all ages — those that have just been created and those that have been around for 120 days and are about to be destroyed. The GHb level in that sample will, therefore, reflect the average blood glucose concentrations of that individual for the last 120 days.

The formation of GHb is fairly slow, and rapid changes in blood glucose levels are averaged out. Normal, non-diabetics will have GHb values between 4 and 8%. Diabetics will typically have GHb concentrations between 8 and 24%. Obviously, the more out of control the diabetic has been, the greater the GHb value. While not typical, it is not impossible for diabetics, especially the Type II, to keep their GHb levels at the top of, or just above, the normal range.

The GHb value has been compared to the batting average of a baseball player. It tells you how well the player has batted during the entire season, but it does not tell you how he batted in the last game[37].

The story behind the discovery of the GHb assay is rather confusing but interesting. It is important to understand the history of the development of this test because there are still many who misuse the terms involved. It started in the late 1950's when two different research groups were passing solutions of hemoglobin through ion exchange columns. The resin in the columns had an electrical charge, and the different hemoglobin variants were held back by the resin to different degrees. Since the charge on the hemoglobin molecule depends on the amino acids in the globin chains, the researchers were using this technique to look for new hemoglobin variants. In addition to the normal Hb A, they found the two fractions that they designated Hb $A_1$ and Hb $A_2$. The second is the normal hemoglobin variant that consists of two alpha and two delta chains. The nature of the first fraction was unknown.

The $A_1$ fraction formed approximately 7% of the total hemoglobin. Additional studies later indicated that $A_1$ is not actually a pure substance. It could be further separated by ion exchange columns into three fractions: Hb $A_{1a}$, $A_{1b}$, and $A_{1c}$.

Then in 1968 Dr. Samuel Rahbar at Tehran University Hospital reported that in a survey of blood samples taken from patients he found two with an unusual variant[38]. Dr. Rahbar was using an electrophoresis technique similar to that used by Linus Pauling to detect Hb S. However, instead of using a liquid solution in which to perform the separation, Dr. Rahbar used a solid

---

37 D. Goldstein, J. Valuck and L. Hazelwood, "The Test That Never Forgets," *Diabetes Forecast* 38(1): 35, Jan/Feb 1985.

38 S. Rahbar, "An abnormal hemoglobin in red cells of diabetics," *Clin Chem Acta* 22:296-298, 1968.

material made from starch. The starch was formed into a slab through which the hemoglobin can move when subjected to an electric current. Differently charged hemoglobins will migrate at different rates, and many new hemoglobin variants have been discovered by electrophoresis.

In his search for hemoglobin variants using starch gel electrophoresis, Dr. Rahbar screened 1,200 blood samples that came into his lab from patients in the hospital. Two of the 1,200 samples contained a hemoglobin variant that moved through the starch gel faster than the normal Hb A. This fast moving fraction accounted for about 10% of the total hemoglobin in these patients.

Upon further investigation Dr. Rahbar learned that both these patients had diabetes. Analysis of the hemoglobin of other individuals with diabetes revealed the presence of this same fast moving fraction. Additional studies by Dr. Rahbar (while at the Albert Einstein College of Medicine in New York) and others indicated that this diabetic hemoglobin is the same as that Hb $A_{1c}$ reported earlier.

Studies of the structure of Hb $A_{1c}$ indicated that it was a normal hemoglobin A molecule with a glucose attached to the end of the beta chain. In non-diabetic individuals the level of $A_{1c}$ is 3-6%. It is the major component of the total Hb $A_1$ fraction. The two remaining fractions, $A_{1a}$ and $A_{1b}$, together form about 2% of total hemoglobin. In a diabetic the level of $A_{1c}$ can increase up to 9-10% if the blood glucose control is very poor. As the average blood glucose concentration drops, the $A_{1c}$ value decreases until it approaches the normal range.

Clinical scientists and physicians soon realized that this assay could be used as the much needed monitor for long-term blood glucose control. By 1977 there were commercial products on the market to allow clinical labs to run the assay routinely. The earliest kits actually measured Hb $A_1$. There were two reasons for this. In the first place, the techniques for measuring $A_{1c}$ alone took about 24 hours. It was too long, complicated and expensive for the regular laboratory. The Hb $A_1$ test could be done in one hour with materials costing about $1.50. In the second place, studies indicated that, whatever their actual structure and origin, the concentration of the combined fraction, Hb $A_{1a+b}$, also elevates as average blood glucose levels increase.[39] (See Figure

---

39 B. Gonen, A. H. Rubenstein, H. Rochman, S. P. Tanega, and D. L. Horwitz, "Haemoglobin A1: An indicator of the metabolic control of diabetic patients," *The Lancet,* Oct. 8, 1977, pp. 734-736.

38.) This implied that total Hb $A_1$ could be used to monitor diabetics with the same degree of accuracy as a pure Hb $A_{1c}$ test.

**Figure 38. Changes in Hb $A_1$ Fractions**

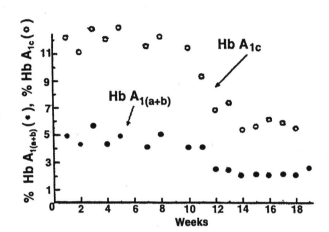

With the advent of a method to measure long-term blood glucose control it became possible to assess the relationship between glucose levels and vascular complications. The National Institutes of Health organized a Diabetes Control and Complications Trial to study diabetes and determine the importance of control in reducing complications. The study was originally intended to last for 10 years, but the results were so clear that it was stopped after 7. The patients were divided into two groups: one received "standard" care; the other received very intensive care — their diet and medications were monitored very closely in an attempt to keep the glucose levels as close to the normal range as possible.

The theory behind the study was that reduced blood glucose levels would be reflected by lowered Hb $A_{1c}$ values[†] and would translate into reduced vascular complications in the diabetics. After 7 years of following the

---

[†] Hb A1c measurements were used because it was, at the time of the start of the DCCT, the best choice for accurate and reproducible results among the labs involved in the study.

members of the study group it became obvious that Hb $A_{1c}$ values less than 7.2% (where normal is less than 6.0%) meant no abnormal development of vascular complications. There is, however, one drawback. Tight control of blood glucose increases the risk of hypoglycemia, which occurs when blood glucose levels fall <u>below</u> normal. Mild hypoglycemia produces confusion and shakiness. More extreme cases can result in loss of consciousness, coma or convulsions. Young diabetics were particularly prone to hypoglycemia because of their active lifestyles, eating habits, and changing bodies. In general, there is a real advantage to maintaining blood glucose control as close to normal as is possible. However, the diabetic's age, physical condition, etc., must be taken into consideration. Higher levels of glucose may be tolerated during certain periods in life in order to reduce the number of hypoglycemic episodes.

This assay has been called by many names: $A_{1c}$, $A_1$, fast hemoglobin, diabetic hemoglobin, glucohemoglobin, glycosylated hemoglobin, GHb, and glycohemoglobin. The terms were all used synonymously although even from the beginning they were not all equivalent.

Even more confusion about the test was created around 1980-1981 when two important observations were made:

1. Hb $A_{1c}$ is not a pure fraction. Only about 75% of it has a glucose attached to the end of the beta chain. The other 25% consists of some other post-translational variants that have the same charge as the glycosylated version and so come out in the same fraction when separated by ion exchange chromatography.

2. Use of a different type of chromatographic resin, called an affinity resin, revealed that there are more glycohemoglobins than just those found in $A_{1c}$. There appear to be sites other than the end of the beta chain where glucose can attach itself to hemoglobin.

Using the affinity column assay scientists found that 4-8% of a normal, non-diabetic's hemoglobin is glycosylated. In diabetes, the glycosylated hemoglobin (GHb) level can rise to as high as 24%. These new discoveries created even more confusion in an already confusing field. Regardless of the complications of the test and the turmoil concerning the proper name by which to call it, the most important question has always been: Does it make any difference for the patient which test is used to monitor diabetes?

For most people it will not make any difference if the lab uses Hb $A_{1c}$, Hb $A_1$, or GHb. As long as the physicians measures the same substance each time, any changes in blood glucose control will be reflected by measuring any of these three substances. It is only important to remember that the numbers are not interchangeable and each has its own scale of values. For example, a normal Hb $A_{1c}$ is 4%, and someone with 8% would be a diabetic in fairly poor control. On the other hand, a GHb value of 8% would be normal while 16% is elevated.

The problem arises for somewhere between 4 and 10% of the population. The biggest complication occurs in people with hemoglobin variants. Assume a diabetic has sickle-cell trait and doesn't know it. Also, assume that 50% of the hemoglobin is Hb A and 50% is Hb S. The glucose in the blood will react equally with A and S. However, the Hb $A_{1c}$ test is specific for $A_{1c}$. It does not measure the similar compound produced when S reacts with glucose. If the Hb $A_{1c}$ value for the diabetic were 4%, the physician might assume the person were in good control. After all, 4% is in the normal range. Yet, the GHb test would probably be about 16% because it measures all the glycosylated hemoglobin regardless of the variants present. The GHb test would warn the physicians that this person is not in good control.

By using the GHb test, physicians do not have to worry about the presence of hemoglobin variants. The test is not complicated by them. But the $A_{1c}$ test will give misleadingly low values if it is not known that the individual has a variant.

Diabetics who are pregnant are particularly concerned with blood glucose control. If they are not in good control, there can be complications with their pregnancy and with the development of the fetus. If the pregnant diabetic is monitored with Hb $A_{1c}$ or Hb $A_1$, and she has a hemoglobin variant, the physician may think she is in good control when, in fact, she is not. The GHb test would give a more accurate indication of her degree of blood glucose control.

There is at least one case reported in the medical literature of a woman who, unknown to herself and her physician, had sickle-cell trait. She also had diabetes, but appeared to be in good control using an Hb $A_1$ test. She had had two pregnancies end with spontaneous abortions – a frequent problem among pregnant diabetics in poor control. Then her physicians ordered the GHb test and found she was not in good control. They also found that she had sickle-cell trait. Her insulin was adjusted, and the third pregnancy resulted in a healthy baby[40].

Physicians working with black diabetics may be aware of the complications due to hemoglobin variants, but few think about this problem with whites of northern European ancestry. They are not routinely tested for variants, and usually only one in 300 has a variant. It is possible for some people with diabetes to go for years under the false assumption they are in good control according to an $A_{1c}$ or $A_1$ test when, in fact, they are in poor control. The result would be an increase in those long term complications to diabetes already mentioned: poor circulation in the feet, problems with vision that may lead to blindness, cardiovascular problems, and deterioration of the kidneys.

Thus far the GHb and Hb $A_1$ fractions are the only post-translational variants studied to any extent. It is possible that in the future the measurement of other variants may help us to understand the chemistry of the blood in both normal and abnormal conditions. There is already some research on one post-translational variant that may help monitor kidney function and another that may measure alcohol consumption and indicate if a person is an alcoholic.

---

40 P. Merrill and S. Trupin, "Hemoglobin A1c levels and variant hemoglobins," *Am J Obstet and Gyn* 149(1):88-89, May 1, 1984.

# Chapter 10

# WEREWOLVES, LEAD POISONING, AND KING GEORGE III

Most of our knowledge about hemoglobin concerns the globin chains and variations in their production. Both normal components and abnormal variants of hemoglobin are the result of alterations in the amino acid sequences in the globin chains. Thalassemias are the result of underproduction of globin chains. However, the other partner molecule in the system should not be forgotten. While there are no genetic variants of the heme molecule, there are both inherited and acquired disorders relating to the biosynthesis of heme. These disorders, known generally as porphyrias, result in the over- or underproduction of heme or in the overproduction of byproducts created during the manufacture of heme.

The heme molecule is actually produced in two places in the body: in the developing red cell and in the liver. While 80% of the heme produced in the body goes into the manufacture of hemoglobin, 20% is incorporated into other molecules. Heme is found in myoglobin, the single heme-globin unit that transports oxygen inside cells, in catalase, an important enzyme in the body, and in cytochrome, a molecule important in the transport of energy.

Porphyrias are disorders related to the production of heme. If it occurs in the developing red cell it is an erythropoietic porphyria. Hepatic porphyrias, on the other hand, occur in the liver. Porphyrias may be either inherited or acquired disorders. Rather than try to cover the complete range of porphyrias, some of which are very rare, we will cover only a few of the major types.

To understand the molecular basis of porphyrias it is first necessary to review again the general pathway used by the body to synthesize heme. Figure 29 in Chapter 5 presents a general outline of the biosynthesis of heme. It may look very complicated at first glance, but there are really only a few basic concepts to remember.

The body does not manufacture heme the same way it synthesizes globin chains. Heme is not a protein. There is no specific DNA sequence that codes for the arrangement of atoms in the heme molecule. Instead, the genetic code carries information for the manufacture of a group of enzymes that are responsible for the manufacture of heme. These enzymes are proteins that are each designed to promote one specific step in the sequence of reactions that result in the production of a heme. The enzymes are not part of the final molecules; they only ensure that the correct molecules come together in the right way to form the desired end product.

The first step in the production of heme is the formation of ALA (aminolevulinic acid). This is an extremely important reaction because it is thought to be the rate controlling step for manufacturing heme. Two small molecules, succinic acid and glycine, are first activated. The succinic acid is attached to coenzyme A and glycine to pyridoxal phosphate. Both of these activating substances take part in the reaction but are not part of the final molecule, ALA. The enzyme ALA synthetase coordinates and promotes the reaction between the activated succinic acid and the activated glycine that results in the formation of ALA. The net result is that the four-carbon succinic acid and the two-carbon glycine have been joined to form a five carbon molecule. One carbon atom is lost as carbon dioxide in the process.

In the next stage, two ALA molecules in the presence of ALA dehydrase, another enzyme, join to form a cyclic compound, PBG. One molecule of water is given off in the process, which is why the enzyme is called a *dehydrase*.

Another group of enzymes cause four PBG molecules to combine to form uroporphyrinogen. Additional enzymatic reactions modify the molecular side groups attached to the large four-ring molecule. During this process it becomes first a coproporphyrinogen, then a protoporphyrinogen, and, finally, a porphyrin. In the last step the enzyme heme synthetase inserts an iron atom into the central cavity formed by the four-ring complex, and the result is heme.

In summary: through the action of enzymes two small molecules are joined to make a longer molecule, two of the longer molecules are shaped into a ring molecule, four ring molecules are combined and changes made in the side groups attached to them, and, finally, iron is added to make heme. Many steps and intermediate products have been ignored. For our discussions it is only important to understand the basic pathway.

Porphyrias are the result of some disruption in this synthetic process. These disruptions can result in the overproduction of intermediates or in the production of by-products to this process. They can be the result of an inherited inborn error of metabolism, or they can be caused by exposure to some environmental factor.

The best known example of an acquired porphyria is lead poisoning. Lead has been used by human societies for over 2,000 years, and it continues to play an important part in many industrial processes and consumer products. Although its toxic properties are well known, there are so many opportunities for exposure to lead that occurrences of lead poisoning, especially in children, are still frequent.

Lead is a very attractive material to work with because it is one of the softest of the common metals and can be easily melted and shaped. In addition, many lead compounds are colorful and make excellent additives in paints, dyes, and ceramic glazes. The Romans formed lead into water pipes and then melted it with tin to make a solder to join the pipes. In the Middle Ages artists started using lead strips to make their stained glass windows.

During the 19th century manufacturers began to rely heavily on lead compounds to give paints color, to make them more durable, and to make them spread easier. White lead, a mixture of lead carbonate and lead hydroxide, has been used as a paint pigment for over 2,000 years. Lead monoxide gives paint a yellow tint, while lead oxide makes it red.

At present the major use for lead is in storage batteries like those used to start automobile and truck engines. It is also used as sheathing for electrical cables, to make bullets and shot, in radiators, and to produce weights for numerous applications. Lead's high density makes it an excellent shield for people working around X-rays and radioactive substances.

In the 1920s gasoline companies began to add tetraethyl lead to their products to make them burn better in automobile engines. The lead itself is not consumed in the process, and auto emissions have dumped an estimated 30 million tons of lead into the environment. The U.S. and other countries have since passed laws to remove lead additives from fuels.

In 1897 two Australian physicians, A.J. Turner and James Gipson, traced the cause of some cases of unexplained illnesses in some of their younger patients to lead in the paint on the porches of the children's houses. In 1920 Australia banned the use of lead in paint, and many other countries have done the same since then. Although it is seldom used in paints today, lead-based paints are still a problem. Many houses and children's toys with lead paint on them are still around.

The symptoms of overexposure to lead are varied. They are not the same in every individual. Lead poisoning may be accompanied by anemia, dizziness, constipation, and colic. It can damage the liver, the kidneys, and tissues in the nervous, reproductive, cardiovascular, and gastrointestinal systems. There is good evidence that lead can retard both physical and intellectual development. Lead can apparently impair a child's ability to learn and reason. Studies indicate that children who suffered from overexposure to lead in early years will have lower IQ's.

Children are more susceptible to the effects of lead poisoning than adults. High levels of lead in children can produce, along with the other symptoms already mentioned, disorders related to the central nervous system (e.g., headaches, visual problems, irritability, and behavioral problems). Serious cases can lead to coma or convulsions. In adults the symptoms most often seen are abdominal pains, constipation, and weakness. But lead definitely has its greatest toxicity in growing bodies, and children will retain up to 50% of the lead they ingest. Adults, in contrast, retain up to 10%.

Some children ingest the lead by putting paint chips in their mouth or chewing on toys or woodwork painted with lead paint. However, the major sources of exposure for both children and adults is the dust created during the renovation, remodeling or repainting of older homes.

Other sources of lead include automobile exhausts and smokestack emissions from certain industrial processes. Lead may also be found in drinking water as a result of leaching from lead pipes, from solder used on copper pipes, or from some plumbing fixtures. The solder that has been used to seal cans may contain lead and may contaminate the food, especially if the contents are acidic. Dinnerware with ceramic glaze made from lead compounds can sometimes be a source of lead poisoning when the glazes have been improperly fired or prepared. Food may also become contaminated if stored in lead crystal for long periods.

Many countries have recognized the dangers of lead toxicity and have taken measures to remove as much as possible from the environment. However, people must be cautious when working with older painted materials and with products produced in areas of the world where there is less concern about consumer health and safety. In some countries lead solder in food cans, lead compounds in paint, and lead additives in gasoline are still permitted. Every year 3.2 million tons of lead are extracted from mines and 5.5 million tons are refined. The difference represents the amount recycled each year. Lead poisoning will be with the earth's population for many years to come.

Lead poisoning affects several areas of the body's metabolism, including the production of heme. Excess levels of lead interfere with two important enzymes in the synthetic pathway for heme. In each case the activity of the enzymes is reduced and there is an accumulation of excess precursor molecules. First, lead decreases the activity of ALA dehydrase. Unused ALA accumulates and will appear in the urine of individuals with lead poisoning. In addition, lead blocks the last step in the production of heme — the insertion of iron into the protoporphyrin. Excess protoporphyrin accumulates in the red cell and can react with zinc atoms (which are in the red cell naturally for other purposes). This results in the production of zinc protoporphyrin (ZnPP), and measurement of ZnPP in the blood is one of the diagnostic tests for lead poisoning.

The lead that is taken in through the lungs or the gastrointestinal tract will end up in several parts of the body. Some will be found in the red cells. When the red cells are destroyed, the lead is excreted in the bile and removed with the feces. Some lead in the blood remains outside the red cells and is handled like calcium. It is deposited in bones. Lead will be found in most body tissues, and it appears in high concentrations in hair. Small amounts will be excreted in the urine. However, in general the body does not have a natural process for removing excess lead very efficiently. If exposure to the source of lead poisoning is halted, it takes several years for the lead content of the body to return to normal.

Porphyria due to lead poisoning is the most commonly seen form of acquired porphyria. Other materials can also induce porphyria. Some insecticides, fungicides, and drugs may produce, among other symptoms, problems in the production of heme. In 1960 there was an outbreak of a porphyria-like disorder in Turkey. People were experiencing blistering of exposed skin, changes in skin pigmentation, scarring, enlarged livers, and red

coloring in their urine. It was discovered that these symptoms were the result
of the exposure of a large number of people to the hexachlorobenzene that was
being used locally as a fungicide to treat wheat.

There are also genetic disorders that cause porphyrias. In some of the
genetic porphyrias there is production of four-ring byproducts and
accumulation of porphyrins in the blood. Some of these ring compounds can
absorb light, resulting in skin sensitive to sunlight. This photosensitivity can
cause a burning discomfort in the individual. Any slight mechanical injury
can produce abrasions, blisters, swellings, and scarring of the skin. After
several years those parts of the skin most exposed to sunlight, the head and
hands, could be covered with scar tissue. Shaving any part of the body would
be very difficult and painful. Anyone with this condition would almost
certainly avoid contact with other people, who would stare at him and find his
strange appearance repulsive. He would also tend to stay out of the sun as
much as possible to avoid the discomfort and pain. Such a person would seem
to many people to be inhuman. The scarred, hairy skin condition might be
interpreted as "wolf-like." A person with a disorder like this could easily be
viewed by others as a half man, half beast demon that hides from the world,
moves only in the night, and does evil things. Unfortunately, in addition to
these physical complications, the excess of heme precursors and by-products
in the blood can lead to neurological problems, mental instability, and
insanity. Legends and tradition about werewolves may simply be the result of
people who have inherited a porphyria before modern medicine made it
possible to understand and partially treat such symptoms.

Porphyrias may have also played an important part in European and
American history. Sir Theodore Lurquet de Mayerne was a French doctor
who served as court physician to James I of England. The doctor kept such
careful records of the King's health and so well described his symptoms when
he was ill that in 1969 two British physicians and medical historians, Ida
Macalpine and Richard Hunter, concluded that James I suffered from a
porphyria[41]. Looking into original records, letters, reports and private diaries
from the periods under study, they were able to trace this genetic disorder
through 500 years and 15 generations of the Royal Houses of Stuart, Tudor,
Hanover, and Brandenberg-Prussia. Although it is difficult to translate the

---

41 Ida Macalpine and Richard Hunter. *George III and the Mad-Business*. The Penguin
    Press, London, 1969.

medical jargon of previous ages into modern terms, and the symptoms of the disease would vary significantly from person to person, there are far too many similarities in illnesses among these people to just be attributed to chance. Those who inherited the porphyria gene typically suffered from pains and weakness in their limbs, color in their urine, a sensitivity to sunlight that often resulted in rashes or a burning sensation on the skin, sweating, fast pulses, sleeplessness, nausea, constipation, and feelings of oppression in the chest. The symptoms would come and go to varying extents and would sometimes be accompanied by mental and emotional problems.

James I (1566-1625) was King of England from 1603 to 1625. He was also James VI, King of Scotland, from 1567 to 1625. Although he had not grown up under her care, he knew that his mother, Mary Queen of Scots (1542-1587), had suffered from attacks of excruciating pain, vomiting, painful lameness, fits and mental disturbances. He told his physician that he had the same disorder his mother had had. James' son, Henry, died at the age of 18 with symptoms suggestive of porphyria. Queen Ann (1665-1714), the great granddaughter of James I, had 17 unsuccessful pregnancies. None of her three children survived her. Records indicate she suffered from "gouty" problems all her life and finally died in a coma at the age of 49.

One of James' granddaughters married Ernst August, Elector of Hanover. Their son became George I, bringing the House of Hanover to the English throne, and their daughter married Frederick I, King of Prussia. Frederick's son, Frederick Wilhelm I, and grandson, Frederick the Great (1712-1786) were both stricken with disorders that appear to be porphyria.

In particular, George III, grandson of George I, was King of England from 1760 to 1820. He ruled during the American Revolution. In 1765 he was very ill with a violent cough, hoarseness, fever, a fast pulse, tiredness and insomnia. He recovered, but the same problems returned in 1788 and were accompanied with dementia (insanity) to such a degree that the Parliament almost passed a bill permitting his son, the Prince of Wales, to rule in the king's name[42]. However, he recovered and continued to rule until 1810, although there were two other short periods of illness and insanity in 1801 and 1804. Then in 1810 he became so hopelessly insane that his son, later George IV, acted as regent until the king died in 1820.

---

42 It is this episode that has been so well portrayed in the 1994 movie *The Madness of King George*.

Macalpine and Hunter suggested in 1969 that George III had inherited porphyria and that metabolic by-products of heme synthesis accumulated in his blood and produced his eventual madness. If George III had been simply a figurehead monarch, his illness would have made little difference in history. However, he took an active part in the government and was a major contributor to the decisions that provoked the American colonists and produced the long conflict that led to the independence of the United States. Exactly to what extent his porphyria affected his judgement is uncertain. While the King's first well defined bout with insanity occurred in 1788, there is no way to determine how the disorder affected his mental state before then. His illness of 1765 lasted several months and was reported as a bad cold, but there is some indication that he also suffered from depression and mental instability.

Certainly he was under a lot of pressure at the time, and it is understandable that he might have been depressed. In the ten years leading up to the American Revolution he had problems in India and Ireland. London was filled with riotous commoners, and he faced the prospect of hostilities from Holland, France, and Spain. Could a more mature, rational monarch have kept the colonies a part of the British empire, or was the split inevitable? No one knows for sure. But it is certain that George III often used poor judgement. He would not listen to those members of Parliament who believed in the validity of the complaints from the American colonists and sought a peaceful reconciliation. Instead, the King favored the sending of troops to the colonies to enforce the laws. The rebellious colonies were a personal affront to his majesty, and his illness may have affected his judgement even before he reached the point where the physicians declared him insane.

George III had 15 children. Four of his sons seem to have inherited the disorder. George IV, who was sick at the time of his father's death in 1820 and who lived only ten more years, suffered many of the physical symptoms of porphyria. George IV married the granddaughter of one of the sisters of Frederick the Great. His wife also had symptoms of porphyria, and it is no surprise that their only child, Charlotte, died at the age of 21 with porphyria-like symptoms.

None of George III's children produced an heir to the throne until Victoria was born in 1819 to the wife of Edward, Duke of Kent, younger brother of George IV. She did not inherit the porphyria gene and had a long, prosperous reign. She did not pass it on to her descendants. (Unfortunately she also carried the trait for the genetic disorder hemophilia and passed it on to her children. In hemophilia the body lacks the ability to produce a molecule that helps clots form in the blood. The DNA defect is located on the X chromosome and can be inherited by females (who are XX) without any effect on their health. It only affects males (who are XY). Victoria gave the gene to one of her sons and two of her daughters. One daughter passed it to her daughter, who married the Russian Czar, Nicholas II, and passed it to their son Alexis.)

The particular variety of porphyria that plagued these royal families appears to be a hepatic porphyria. Neither the red cells nor the bone marrow seem to be affected. It is important to note that the genetics of porphyria are different from those of the hemoglobinopathies. Sickle cell anemia, thalassemias, and other hemoglobinopathies affect the health only when an individual inherits the gene from both parents. Those who are heterozygous (i.e, they have one normal and one abnormal gene) generally have no medical problems. This type of genetic disorder is a *recessive* trait — its presence can be masked by the functioning of the normal gene, but it can be passed on to offspring. Porphyria is a *dominant* trait. The presence of just one abnormal gene will affect the health — the normal gene will not mask the presence of the abnormal one. This means that each child of a person with porphyria has a 50% chance of inheriting the disorder and a 50% chance of receiving two normal genes. If both parents have the trait, as in the case of George IV and his wife, then each child has a 75% chance of having the disorder.

The exact biochemical basis of the porphyrias is not clearly understood. Medical literature on the subject has been mostly limited to descriptions of the symptoms of the various types of porphyrias. There is little knowledge about the exact genetic defect that causes porphyrias. However, it is clear that there are many different types of erythropoietic and hepatic porphyrias. Some are serious; some are mild. Some remain latent until some external agent, like alcohol or barbiturates, provokes an attack.

The majority of porphyrias seem to result in the production of excess amounts of ALA. Since this is the rate-controlling step in the production of heme, it would seem that anything which caused an excess of ALA would lead to overproduction of heme and many of its precursors. There is one mechanism that has been proposed, but not yet totally proven, that could explain many of the porphyrias[43].

As was discussed in Chapter 5, a segment of DNA in the chromosomes carries the genetic code for the manufacture of ALA synthetase. The DNA code is transferred onto a messenger RNA (mRNA) molecule, which is used by the cell to produce the protein ALA synthetase. Another section of DNA produces a protein called an operator that controls the production of the ALA synthetase mRNA. A third DNA section produces a protein called an aporepressor. When there is excess heme present, it reacts with the aporepressor to form a repressor that interferes with the operator and stops the production of the mRNA. This is the cell's feedback mechanism to prevent the overproduction of ALA synthetase. When there is more than enough heme, the excess forms a repressor molecule to stop production of more ALA synthetase. If the level of heme drops, there is less repressor and the operator can reactivate the production of ALA synthetase.

If there were a mutation at the DNA site for the operator such that the repressor molecule could no longer react with it, there would be no mechanism to stop ALA synthetase production. Increased ALA synthetase would result in increased ALA, PBG, etc. In addition, any chemicals that could react with the aporepressor molecule and make it unavailable for formation of repressor with heme would also lead to overproduction of ALA synthetase.

There is some evidence that the above scheme accounts for both some genetic and some acquired porphyrias. This is not the only theory, but it serves as a good illustration of the complexities of the biochemical reactions that occur in cells.

---

43 John Harris and Robert Kellermeyer. *The Red Cell*. Harvard University Press, Cambridge, 1963.

# Chapter 11

# HEMOGLOBIN, GENETICS AND PUBLIC POLICIES

On February 18, 1981, President Nixon addressed the nation with his health message. Among his other proposals he singled out sickle-cell anemia for special attention. He described it as a major health problem in the United States that had been neglected too long and proposed reversing the years of neglect by special government efforts to study the disorder. Up until that time few people, even in the black community, realized the nature and extent of sickle-cell anemia. The government had been spending about one million dollars a year on research into sickle-cell anemia, but there was very little direction or public policy. Suddenly it all changed. Now Congressmen, baseball players, actors, black community leaders, and the news media were calling for a national commitment to find the causes and cures for sickle-cell anemia. President Nixon proposed increasing the budget to $5 million, but by the time the National Sickle Cell Control Act was passed, the Congressional appropriation had risen to $25 million.

The goal of the Act was to "conquer" sickle-cell anemia by the detection, prevention and treatment of the disease on a national level. The money was to be spent for the establishment of sickle-cell centers, for grants supporting research into the causes and possible cures of sickle-cell anemia, and for clinics that would test for sickle-cell anemia and sickle-cell trait and counsel people about the disorder.

While there is no doubt a disease of this magnitude deserved greater public interest and support than it was receiving, there was a great deal of misunderstanding and lack of clear direction in the early stages of the program.

One of the major problems was the misunderstanding, especially among the public, about the differences between those who had sickle-cell anemia and those who merely carried the trait. Although there is no indication that carriers suffer any adverse health problems because they have the trait, there were reportedly cases of discrimination by the uninformed. Doctors were recommending that carriers avoid any situation where low oxygen levels might cause their cells to sickle: mountain climbing, flying, scuba diving, strenuous exercise, etc. The Armed Services refused to let those with the trait engage in certain occupations (like becoming a pilot). As late as 1980 there was still a controversy over the admission of carriers of the sickle-cell trait to the U.S. Air Force Academy. The Air Force contended that the low oxygen environment at high altitudes might cause the cells of an AS individual to sickle. There was, however, no medical evidence to back this up. AS blood could only be made to sickle on a microscope slide when covered by a glass slip that created a zero-oxygen condition. In 1981, under pressure from a lawsuit, the Air Force reversed its policy.

In addition to the misunderstandings, which have the potential of being cleared up in time, there was a great deal of uncertainty as to what our public policy should be. If the government sets up clinics with free testing for sickle-cell trait, what should happen when it is detected? Do the counselors explain the situation and let the carrier decide? Do we want to tell a carrier that he or she should not marry another carrier? What if two carriers are already married? Should the public health policy be to explain the 25% chance of two carriers having a child with sickle-cell anemia but then let the married couple decide? Or should the public try to be more forceful? Should counselors encourage those with the trait not to marry another carrier? If two carriers are married, should they be advised not to have children? After all, there is still a 75% probability that their child will be healthy.

If two carriers marry and have a child, should society encourage testing of the fetus and provide for abortion if the child has sickle-cell anemia? People with sickle-cell anemia usually lead lives filled with pain, suffering and early death. Their birth causes tremendous economic and psychological burdens for the family, for themselves, and for society in general.

Whatever a couple decides to do, there is no doubt that counseling can be effective. For several years there have been programs in Greece, Italy, and Sardinia to screen for beta-thalassemia and to counsel carriers of the trait. The result has been a significant decrease in the incidence of the disorder in those areas where the programs have been implemented.

It is one thing to talk about detection of sickle-cell anemia, but it is quite another problem to decide what is meant by "preventing" a genetic disease. This is a very serious question, but it will eventually have to be answered. There is growing interest in genetic diseases, and there are significant advances in genetic research that will allow us to detect and perhaps cure some genetic diseases. The question of our public policy regarding prevention will soon have to be established.

The National Sickle Cell Control Act was actually the second attempt by society to detect and prevent a genetic disorder. The first experience was less controversial and much less complicated. It involved testing newborns for PKU (phenylketonuria). PKU is a genetic defect wherein the body is unable to produce an enzyme that metabolizes the amino acid phenylalanine. The accumulation of phenylalanine in the body can lead to irreversible mental retardation. However, if the disorder is detected soon after birth, the individual with PKU can be placed on a special diet that contains no phenylalanine. (Those not familiar with this disorder should note the warning labels on foods and beverages containing non-nutritive sweeteners that decompose in the body to phenylalanine.)

In 1961 Dr. Robert Guthrie at Children's Hospital in Buffalo developed a simple test to detect PKU in babies. The test is done using a dried blood sample collected from the newborn by pricking the baby's heel and pressing a few drops of blood on a special piece of paper. Every one of the states in the U.S. has enacted laws that require hospitals, the public health department, or physicians to test for PKU in the first six months of life. Many other countries provide nationwide screening of newborns for PKU. These screening programs for PKU made it possible to reduce the number of people mentally retarded because of PKU. The test is only done after birth, so there was no question of suggesting abortions. It is not yet possible to predict which parents will have a child with PKU, so the question of genetic counseling never arose.

The success of the PKU screening program led to the development of other assays for similar inborn errors of metabolism. Like PKU, these genetic disorders result in the accumulation of unwanted amino acids in the blood. In most cases the consequence is some degree of mental retardation. Fortunately, the fetus with an inborn error in amino acid metabolism is protected by the maternal circulation while in the womb. The accumulation of unwanted amino acids does not start until after birth. Early detection followed by treatment with the appropriate diet will mitigate or prevent problems and permit the affected child to develop normally both physically and mentally.

But, it is very critical that the disorder be detected as soon as possible after birth. A newborn with PKU will have normal levels of phenylalanine at birth; within just a few hours after a baby leaves the womb phenylalanine levels in the blood will start to increase. If the child is not placed on a special, phenylalanine-free diet, signs of developmental delays will start to appear by the age of 6 months. Placing the child on the special diet will prevent mental retardation.

Another common inborn error of metabolism is Maple Syrup Urine Disease (MSUD). Infants with this disorder most often die; those who do survive suffer brain damage and become mentally retarded. Diagnosis within the first few days of life and treatment with a special diet will save the lives of children with MSUD and permit them to develop normally. Homocystinuria and galactosemia are similar to PKU and MSUD. They can be detected by screening newborns and, if found early enough, be treated.

There has been interest in looking at newborns for other disorders in addition to inborn errors of amino acid metabolism. Congenital hypothyroidism (CH) is found in the U.S. population with a frequency three times that of PKU. Infants with CH will become mentally retarded unless treated by a simple medication that replaces the thyroxine not produced in their bodies.

Because of their simplicity and success, the screening programs for PKU and other genetic diseases appear to be well accepted and easily justified on the basis of the savings to society by preventing problems that would be very expensive to handle after the infant grows older. Screening programs have been established by law in every state in the Union. The sickle-cell program, on the other hand, introduced many other considerations that made it more controversial. And, as more genetic screening programs are added, these issues will not disappear. They must be faced.

There is every indication that genetic screening will increase in the future. With the passage of the Sickle-Cell Anemia Control Act there was an upsurge of interest by ethnic groups in their own genetic disorder. U.S. citizens of Italian, Spanish and Portuguese ancestry wanted a similar program for Cooley's anemia (i.e., beta-thalassemia). The Jewish population was interested in research and screening for Tay-Sachs disease, a very serious neurological disorder that is seen in Jews of middle European ancestry.

The Congress soon reformulated the program and in 1976 passed the Genetic Disease Act. This legislation included sickle-cell anemia, Cooley's anemia, Tay-Sachs disease, and any other genetic disorder. While sickle-cell anemia is still the major genetic disorder of interest in the U.S., there are definite programs underway to screen for other conditions.

Sometimes the problems presented are limited by the screening test. If the disorder can't be detected until after birth, as in PKU, the question of genetic counseling for parents and concerns about abortion do not arise. However, advances in medical technology will no doubt soon make possible the prediction of the risk of having children with a genetic disorder and the possibility of detecting these disorders early in the development of the fetus.

At present there is little testing of fetuses for sickle-cell anemia. There are, however, institutions which will test the fetus before 18 weeks old for Cooley's anemia (the homozygous form of beta-thalassemia). This is not done on every fetus, only those at high risk for the disease (i.e., both parents carry the trait). If the test is positive the parents may elect to have an abortion.

In addition to detection and prevention, there is also the question of cure. Should we make an effort to cure serious genetic diseases? The humane answer would be yes, but this will lead society to other problems. "Curing" a genetic disorder usually involves some treatment of the body to make up for the genetic defect. Several possible methods for treating sickle-cell anemia are under investigation. One approach is to introduce into the blood stream a chemical that will react with Hb S and prevent it from sickling. A more promising possibility, and one less dangerous to the patient, is the use of a drug to switch on the production of Hb F. Newborns with sickle-cell anemia do not have a problem with sickling because their main hemoglobin is F. At birth the gene controlling the production of Hb F is turned off, and that controlling the Hb S gene is turned on. As the baby grows its F is gradually replaced with S, and sickling becomes possible. If the adult could turn the F gene back on, the fetal hemoglobin would essentially dilute the S and keep it from sickling.

The use of drugs to prevent sickling directly or to increase the concentration of Hb F could reduce the number of painful crises a person with sickle-cell anemia might experience. The drugs would have to be administered intravenously on a regular basis, but the patient would be able to lead a relatively normal, pain-free life. The disease would not be cured or eliminated, but pain and suffering would be alleviated.

Another approach close to being perfected involves repair of the genetic error in the nucleus of the stem cell. If a foreign stem cell were introduced into the bone marrow, the body would see it as an infection and attack it with its immune system. Therefore, it is best to take a stem cell from the patient, repair it, and then replace it in the marrow. This may sound complicated, but the techniques for doing this are already well developed in the laboratory. It has the potential to "cure" sickle-cell anemia, beta-thalassemia, and any other disorder relayed to the red cells, white cells, or platelets. The basic procedure would be the same in every case:

First, the exact variation in the DNA code that causes the disorder must be determined. A small section of DNA must be synthesized with the corrected nucleotide sequence. The DNA segment is placed in a vector – this could be a virus or a bacterium. Stem cells removed from the patient are cultured with the vector, which infects the cell, carrying with it the correct code. Alternately, there are other methods that might be used to splice out the incorrect code from the stem cell's DNA and patch it with the corrected code.

The repaired cell is then re-implanted in the bone marrow. To insure the survival of the new stem cells, the patient may first be given radiation or chemotherapy to kill all the old stem cells. The new stem cell will grow, divide, and multiply. New blood cells produced from these stem cells will now produce proteins with the correct amino acid sequence.

In all of these cures, whether with drugs or with repaired stem cells, the person still possesses the sickle-cell gene in their germ cells — the cells that will be used to produce children. They can pass the gene on to future generations. Increasing the survival rate and improving the health of people with any genetic disorder will certainly increase the frequency of the disorder in the world.

There are, however, other technological changes that may come to society's rescue. Many people fear the current research with "test tube" babies because they believe it may lead to manipulation of human life — the breeding of people to meet specific standards. While there may be some danger of this, many people overlook the benefits of such technology.

To create a baby in a test tube, the doctor takes a sperm from the male and an ova from the female and allows them to combine in a test tube. The fertilized cell is then transplanted to the mother's womb and allowed to develop as a normal fetus.

If the two people want to have a child but are both carriers of a genetic disease trait, they could have the doctor eliminate fertilized cells that would result in a child with the disease. This procedure would not only give the parents freedom of choice about having a child, but they, and society, could be assured that the child would not suffer from a genetic disease. Even if the disease can be "cured," it would be more economical for everyone and more beneficial for society if the disease could be prevented.

Although many complain that the sickle-cell screening program was not established with a definite public policy in mind, perhaps it's just as well. If the Congress and the people had been forced to consider public policy on abortion for genetic diseases, fetal testing, genetic engineering, etc., they would probably have established narrow and rigid guidelines before all the options were clear and available.

Many people are concerned about genetic screening because of their speculations about the idea that here might be a potential for misuse of genetic information. They tend to forget that genetic screening information is used around the world to save lives. In the United States every state requires that newborns be tested for hemoglobin variants. While it is a general screening for hemoglobin variants, the primary goal is to locate babies with sickle-cell anemia.

The purpose of the screening is not to increase insurance rates or deny jobs to these children. Society is not collecting this information to use against these babies when they grow up. It will be obvious long before adulthood that these children have sickle-cell anemia.

The purpose of the screening is to save lives. Young children with sickle-cell anemia can easily develop life-threatening complications. They often have an enlarged spleen. Because the spleen helps to protect against infections, malfunctions of that organ can help turn a normal bacterial infection into a severe illness. Infections are the major cause of death among children with sickle-cell anemia. Infants as young as 3 months old can develop infections that progress from onset of fever to death in as little as nine hours. The most frequently seen infections in these children are meningitis, pneumonia, and influenza.

If a child is known to have sickle-cell anemia, he or she can be given daily doses of penicillin to combat potential infections. Physicians can educate the parents about the disease, show them how to look for enlargement of the spleen, and stress that they should seek help immediately if the child has a fever.

Before the introduction of newborn screening, fatality rates were as high as 30% among children born with sickle-cell anemia. Almost 1/3 of all children with sickle-cell anemia would die within the first five years of life as a result of bacterial infections or severe anemia. With screening the death rate has dropped significantly[44].

In addition to saving the lives of children with sickle-cell anemia, screening will also detect children with sickle-cell trait. This may help alert unknowing parents that one or both are carriers of the trait. After they have been tested they will know if it is possible that any future child may have the disease.

These serious matters will have to be faced by the public, by the medical community, by legislatures, by courts, and by parents in the near future. To arrive at answers will take an understanding of the genetic disorders involved, an appreciation for the technology available, and a respect for the quality of human life. Those who jump to conclusions on the basis of their prejudices will only retard the progress of human society.

---

44 D. A. Armbruster, "Neonatal hemoglobinopathy screening," *Lab Med*, 21(12): 815-822 (Dec 1990).

# Chapter 12

# A SHORT REVIEW

This book was written to introduce hemoglobin and explain its role in human health. While some prior knowledge of certain topics in chemistry, history, and medicine might have been helpful to the reader, every attempt has been made to introduce and explain new concepts with such care that they could be understood by any interested reader. In fact, a study of hemoglobin is an excellent way to introduce the basics of DNA, RNA, protein synthesis, genetic disorders, respiration, and related topics. Since repetition is one of the key elements in learning new ideas, it would be worthwhile to review and summarize what has been covered.

Historically we arrived at our understanding of hemoglobin through investigations into the nature and function of blood. While ancient civilizations appreciated the importance of blood in life, they did not understand its role. The Greeks and Romans could distinguish between veins and arteries, but they never understood why they were different. While William Harvey is usually credited with publishing the first clear description of the circulation of the blood, his work was preceded and supported by the efforts and discoveries of many others. Servetus, Ibn al-Nofis, and Realdo Colombo had described the pulmonary circulation of the blood. The Italian Cesalpino published a clear description of the complete circulation of the blood 35 years before Harvey's work. Cesalpino also reported that there are small hair-like vessels that he called capillaries connecting the arteries with the veins. Harvey missed that point and thought that tissues contained pores through which the blood passed from the arteries to the veins. Unfortunately, Cesalpino's theological views offended both the Protestants and the Catholics, and his medical work was not given the attention it deserved.

In the eighteenth century Lavoisier demonstrated that the respiration of human beings was a form of controlled combustion: the reaction of oxygen with some fuel. In 1837 Heinrich Gustav Magnus found that blood in the arteries contains more oxygen than that in the veins and that carbon dioxide in the veins comes from the body's tissues. The question then became: are these gases, carbon dioxide and oxygen, simply dissolved in the blood or is there some substance that transports them? It soon became apparent that solubility accounts for only a small percentage of the gases in the blood. There had to be something in the blood responsible for carrying the gases.

Meanwhile several investigators had noted that there is a substance in the blood that would form red crystals. This material could be separated into two components: a clear protein and a red, non-protein material. In 1864 Felix Hoppe-Seyler gave this substance the name hemoglobin and found that it could bind oxygen, but the bond was very weak and the gas could be easily released to the cells. He was also the first to look at the absorption of light by hemoglobin, and he demonstrated its similarity to chlorophyll, the green pigment in plants.

In England G. G. Stokes used Hoppe-Seyler's spectra of hemoglobin to study the changing color of blood. He found that the absorption peaks (and hence, the color) of hemoglobin changes as oxygen is added to or removed from the molecule. This explains why the blood in the veins has a different color from that in the arteries.

Gustav Hüfner published an equation predicting the affinity of hemoglobin for oxygen at various pressures. His resulting curve, however, did not quite fit the true behavior of hemoglobin. It was a better description for the performance of myoglobin, a molecule one-fourth the size of hemoglobin that stores the gas inside the cell. The actual hemoglobin-oxygen curve as described by Hasselbach, Krogh and Bohr differed slightly from that of Hüfner. Their curve indicated that hemoglobin will give up more oxygen to the cells than myoglobin and is thus better suited to transport the gas from the lungs to the tissues.

Simple elemental analysis of the molecule indicated that it contained iron, and iron was known to react readily with oxygen. The possibility that attachment of oxygen to the hemoglobin molecule might occur at the iron was considered, but the change in oxidation states of the metal involved more energy that could be expected in a biological system. How could the iron-oxygen bond be so easily formed and broken? The problem became even more puzzling when James Conant demonstrated in 1923 that the iron in hemoglobin remains in the +2 oxidation state during the complete respiratory cycle: capturing oxygen in the lungs, transporting it through the blood, releasing it to the cells, and returning to the lungs for more. This could not be explained until the structure of hemoglobin had been determined.

The basic formula for hemoglobin was established by Zinofsky in 1885. He found that for each iron atom the hemoglobin molecule contains 712 carbon, 1,130 hydrogen, 214 nitrogen, 243 oxygen, and 2 sulfur atoms. However, he did not know how many iron atoms were in each molecule of hemoglobin. Adair, using osmotic pressure measurements, and Svedberg, working with his newly invented ultracentrifuge, each independently found that hemoglobin has a molecular weight of about 67,000. This implied four irons in each molecule.

Several research groups found that there are two pairs of protein chains in each hemoglobin molecule. The two short chains were called alpha, the two long chains were designated beta. Other scientists found that the non-protein portion of hemoglobin belongs to a class of compounds called porphyrins — flat, disc-shaped molecules with an iron in the center. Max Perutz and his coworkers, using X-ray analysis of hemoglobin crystals, worked for 23 years to determine the three-dimensional arrangement of the atoms.

The hemoglobin molecule is actually four heme-globin units. Each unit has a globin (the protein) and a heme (the porphyrin with an iron in the center). The globin is a long chain of amino acids that is coiled in such a way as to form a small pocket in which the heme sits. One particular amino acid, a histidine, is stationed in back of the iron and pulls it in towards the globin. All four hemes are the same, but two are associated with alpha chains and two with beta. It is the interactions between the four units that make hemoglobin a better transporter of oxygen than myoglobin, which is essentially one heme-globin unit.

In the lungs the oxygen pressure (about 100 mm) in the alveolar sack forces $O_2$ molecules through a thin membrane into the blood stream. One of the excess oxygens attaches itself to a heme and "pops" the iron out of the molecular plane. The motion is translated via movement of the globin to the other heme-globin units in the molecule. The change in the structure of the molecule pushes the other iron atoms out, exposing them to other oxygens in the blood. Thus, once one oxygen has attached itself the rest of the molecule changes shape and readily picks up three more oxygens.

When the globin moves as oxygen is picked up, there are changes in salt bridges between amino acids on adjacent chains. As a result hydrogen ions ($H^+$) are released into the blood. These ions react with the bicarbonate in the blood and form carbonic acid, which quickly decomposes to water and carbon dioxide. There is an increase in carbon dioxide pressure in the blood, causing the gas to pass into the lungs, where it is expelled.

The hemoglobin molecules, packed in the red cells, travel in the blood stream to the various tissues of the body. There, in a low oxygen, high carbon dioxide environment, the process is reversed. The $O_2$ molecules leave the iron and diffuse out of the erythrocyte, through the capillary wall, and into the cells, where they are picked up by myoglobin. Departure of one oxygen causes an iron to pop back into the heme plane. The globin chain moves, forcing other oxygen molecules to be expelled. New salt bridges are formed, hydrogen ions are absorbed, and more carbon dioxide from the cells can dissolve in the blood. The blood returns to the lung to start the cycle over..

The structure of hemoglobin makes it so well suited for the transport of respiratory gases that it has become the major respiratory pigment in living organisms on Earth. The hemoglobin molecules differ slightly from species to species in the exact amino acid sequences of the globin chains, but they all have essentially the same structure and work in the same way. Nature has not yet found a better way to carry oxygen to the cells of large animals and remove the poisonous carbon dioxide produced by metabolic processes. Humanity's efforts to find a substitute have not been very successful either. There is a serious need for an artificial substitute for blood. It is often needed in accidents, trauma cases, medical treatments that destroy red cells, surgeries where there is a loss of blood, etc. Transfusion of human blood can now be accomplished safely and routinely, but there is growing concern about the transmission of undetected pathogens. The best candidates for replacing blood transfusions are animal hemoglobins or modified human hemoglobins that cannot be destroyed by the body's normal processes.

Hemoglobin is not found free in the blood. It is found in the red cells, which form about 50% of the total volume of the blood. These cells are produced in the bone marrow from stem cells. A chemical signal is produced in the kidneys when there is a slight decrease in oxygen being delivered there.

This signal, erythropoietin, starts the process by which a stem cell is converted to eight red cells. As they mature, the red cells manufacture hemoglobin using the genetic information contained in the nucleus of the cell. When it is ready to be placed in the blood stream, the red cell is essentially a bag of hemoglobin molecules with no purpose other than gas transport. The nuclear material is destroyed, so the cell cannot continue to produce proteins once it is in the blood. A typical red cell will last for 120 days before it is destroyed by the spleen or by macrophages in the blood.

The maturing red cell uses the genetic information on chromosomes 16 and 11 to make the alpha and beta chains. The DNA molecules carry the information on the exact sequence of amino acids needed to produce a specific protein. This code is found in the sequence of nucleotides, G, C, A, and T, on the DNA molecule. The red cell transcribes this code to a messenger RNA molecule, which carries it to the ribosome in the cell's cytoplasm. At the ribosome the code is translated to the correct sequence of amino acids needed to produce a specific protein. Transfer RNAs have an amino acid at one end and the corresponding nucleotide code at the other. The ribosome matches the code on the mRNA with the appropriate tRNA and links the amino acids together. The tRNA returns to pick up more amino acids and the mRNA is destroyed.

Since the heme is not a protein, it must be produced in a different manner. The cell synthesizes a series of enzymes that promote a sequence of reactions that result in the creation of the heme molecule. Finally, each heme is surrounded by one of the globin chains, and four heme-globin units are combined to form the completed molecule.

The hemoglobin molecule with two alpha and two beta chains is the normal adult hemoglobin, Hb A. There are actually several normal components of hemoglobin that differ slightly from each other in the exact sequence of amino acids in the globin chains. There are embryonic and fetal hemoglobins formed during the development of a human being from single cell to newborn baby. These hemoglobin components all have the same heme, and each has two alpha (or alpha-like) globins and two beta (or beta-like) globins. Genetic information for all the alpha and alpha-like chains is found on chromosome 16. The remaining chains are coded in chromosome 11. In the majority of adults there will be 97% Hb A, about 1% Hb F, and about 2% Hb $A_2$.

We don't really know the reasons for all these components. However, it would appear that the fetus needs a hemoglobin with a greater affinity for oxygen than the mother's. Thus, when Hb F, with two alpha and two gamma chains, in the baby's blood passes near the mother's Hb A in the placenta, the F can pull some of the oxygen from the A. This provides the fetus with the energy needed to grow and develop. After birth the infant's stem cells turn off the production of F and increase the production of Hb A. By the age of one year there is little F remaining, and Hb A is the major component.

There does not appear to be any particular reason for the Hb $A_2$ in our bodies. It may simply be left over from our evolutionary past. It contains two alpha and two delta chains and seems no have no particular influence on human health. However, abnormally high concentrations of Hb $A_2$ (greater than 3.5%) are a good diagnostic indicator for beta-thalassemia trait.

Hemoglobin plays such an important role in the normal functioning of the human body that a measurement of its concentration is one of the best general indicators of a person's health. Typical hemoglobin levels are 14-18 g/100 ml for men and 12-16 g/100mL for women. Any significant decline in the amount of hemoglobin in the blood is an anemia. Anemias may be caused by many different factors, but the most common are nutritional deficiencies. Poor diets lacking in iron, folic acid, amino acids, etc., leave the body unable to produce the red cells and the hemoglobin it needs.

Pernicious anemia results when vitamin $B_{12}$ in the diet cannot be absorbed into the body. The mucous membrane lining the stomach is not able to produce the molecule that is used to form the complex needed to bring in the $B_{12}$. Without this vitamin the red cells cannot grow and divide.

Aplastic anemia occurs when the bone marrow is not able to produce adequate numbers of red cells. The causes of this disorder are not always known, but it frequently is the result of exposure to toxic substances, especially during the radiation and chemical therapies used on cancer patients.

Some anemias are due to hereditary defects. G-6-PD is an enzyme in the red cells. A deficiency in this enzyme is the result of a genetic condition that is found widely in Mediterranean peoples. Certain substances in the diet may cause red cells to clump together and break down if the individual has G-6-PD deficiency. This rupturing, or lysing, of the red cells turns the urine red and decreases the amount of hemoglobin in the blood. The fava, or Italian broad, bean (especially when lightly cooked) was found to cause hemolytic anemia in people with G-6-PD deficiency. The Greek philosopher and mathematician

Pythagoras might have had this disorder. It would explain why he forbade his followers to eat beans. Many drugs, including anti-malarials, can also trigger hemolytic anemia. Perhaps 100 million people have this disorder.

Anemias can also be the result of underproduction of globin chains. These disorders, called thalassemias, are named by the affected globin chain. Beta-thalassemia is very common among people of Mediterranean ancestry (Italians, Greeks, Sicilians, Spaniards, Turks, North Africans, etc.). A person who inherits the beta-thalassemia gene from one parent is heterozygous for the condition. They might have a slight reduction in hemoglobin level, but they generally suffer no adverse health problems. However, the homozygous condition, where the gene is received from both parents, is very serious. Approximately 1,000 people in the U.S. suffer from this condition.

The varieties of alpha-thalassemia are more complicated because there are four genes directing the production of alpha chains. Disorders can come from the deletion or inactivation of one, two, three, or all four genes. The last condition, hydrops fetalis, is not compatible with life, and the baby is usually stillborn. Hydrops fetalis is a very serious public health issue in Southeast Asia, particularly in Thailand. Lack of one or two alpha genes has little effect on the person's health. The absence of three alpha genes results in an overproduction of beta chains, which can combine to form Hb H, an unstable hemoglobin molecule with four beta chains. People with Hb H disease are usually anemic.

Thalassemias are due to one of two genetic conditions: either sections coding for the globin chain have been deleted or there are errors in sections of the code that produce proteins that control the rate of chain production. The majority of alpha-thalassemias are attributed to missing genes; most beta-thalassemias have a complete code for the beta chain but have other errors that affect the amount of beta chain produced.

When there is a single point mutation in the DNA code, and the result is a substitution of one amino acid for another when the chain is manufactured, the result is a hemoglobin variant. In particular, when the sixth amino acid in the beta chain is valine, rather than the normal lysine, the variant is Hb S. This variant, when produced by both genes, is the cause of sickle-cell anemia. This one alteration in the amino acid sequence permits the molecule to crystallize in a low oxygen environment. These crystals grow so long that they distort the red cell, causing it to plug the entrances in capillaries and small blood vessels.

Approximately one out of ten black people of African ancestry in the United States carries the Hb S trait. It does not create a health problem for them, but if two carriers have children, there is a 25% chance that each child will inherit the gene from both parents. This homozygous condition, sickle-cell anemia, can be very serious. The plugging of the blood vessels can cause pain, especially in the joints, and will keep oxygen from the tissues. There is a reduced ability to fight infections, particularly in young children.

There are over 700 known hemoglobin variants. Some, like hemoglobins S, E, and C, are found in millions of people. Other have been found in only a few families and seem to be very rare. There is a very high incidence of Hb E in Asia, and it may, in fact, be the most common hemoglobin variant in the world. The homozygous form, Hb E disease, results in some anemia, but it is not as serious as sickle-cell anemia.

Hemoglobin variants come from a mutation in the genetic code. They are produced when the code is translated in the ribosome. Any changes to the hemoglobin molecule after this are thus post-translational. The best known, and most important, post-translational variants are the glycohemoglobins (GHb). Glucose in the blood attaches itself slowly, and irreversibly, to hemoglobin at several points along the globin chains. This reaction occurs in every person and continues throughout the 120 day life of the red cell. If a person's average blood glucose levels are higher than normal, as they may be in diabetes, the concentration of GHb will increase. Hence, measurement of GHb levels can be used to monitor the treatment of diabetics. Any changes in blood glucose control is reflected very slowly in changes in GHb. Improved blood glucose control will reduce the long-term complications that may occur in diabetics: vision problems, poor circulation, kidney disorders, etc.

Most of the genetic disorders related to hemoglobin involve the globin chains. There are no known variants of the other partner, the heme. However, there are inherited and acquired disorders related to the production of heme and some of its precursors. These are the porphyrias. The most common acquired porphyria is lead poisoning. Genetic porphyrias have a wide variety of symptoms and are generally rather rare. Typical symptoms include colored urine, sensitivity to sunlight, scarring of tissues exposed to the sun (e.g., hands and face), pain in the joints, constipation, general malaise, and, in extreme cases, bouts of insanity. It may be that legends about werewolves are based on true incidents of individuals with a porphyria who avoided sunlight, had scarred, hairy faces and hands, and behaved irrationally. It also appears that a porphyria gene passed through several English and European royal families for the last 500 years. There is strong evidence that the madness of George III, king of England during the American Revolution, was caused by an inherited porphyria.

Much of the modern research on hemoglobin is the result of an increased funding for the study of sickle-cell anemia. No cure has been found for the disease, but there are several treatments that show some promise of reducing the pain and suffering. One technique would use a drug to increase the amount of Hb F in people with sickle-cell anemia. The Hb F essentially dilutes the Hb S and keeps it from sickling. There has also been a significant increase in screening both adults and newborns for Hb S trait and sickle-cell anemia. It is especially important to identify babies who are homozygous for Hb S. They have trouble fighting infections and can die from sicknesses that are simply a normal childhood experience for other children. Every state has a program to screen all newborns for hemoglobin variants. Children with sickle-cell disease are monitored carefully and usually given antibiotics to prevent infections.

The screening for sickle-cell anemia is part of larger programs that look for genetic disorders that can lead to irreversible mental retardation if not treated soon after birth. All babies born in the United States are routinely tested for phenylketonuria, galactosemia, thyroid dysfunctions and similar disorders where early detection and treatment will save lives and prevent developmental problems.

Knowledge about hemoglobin will help people make more informed decisions about public health issues and about their own health. It should also create a greater appreciation for the complexities of life. This book has presented only a basic introduction to this fascinating, and extremely important, molecule. Those who would like to learn more about the genetics, biochemistry, history, and politics of hemoglobin will find some suggestions in "Additional Readings."

# GLOSSARY
## OF UNCOMMON WORDS AND ACRONYMS

### PRONUNCIATION SYMBOLS

ă as **a** in hat       ō as **o** in tone
ā as **a** in pay       ô as **a** in paw
ĕ as **e** in bet       ŏ as **o** in pot
ē as **e** in me        ü as **oo** in boot
i as **i** in pit       ə as **a** in about
ī as **i** in file

**alveolus** (ăl-vē´ə-ləs), the small air sac in the lung where gas exchange takes place.

**amino acid** (ə-mē´nō ăs´id), an organic compound containing both an amine (-NH₂) and a carboxylic acid (-COOH).

**anticodon** (ăn´ti-kō-don), a triplet of nucleotide bases in transfer RNA that matches with a complementary triplet in messenger RNA.

**codon** (kō´dŏn), a group of three nucleotides that form the code for one amino acid.

**DNA, deoxyribonucleic acid** (dē-ŏk´sē-rī´bō-nü´klā´ik as´id), a helical molecule consisting of alternating phosphate and sugar groups to which are attached the nucleotides that carry the genetic code.

**electrophoresis** (i-lk´tro-fə-r´sis), a laboratory technique that separates proteins based on charge differences. (Although not discussed in this book, the technique can also be used to separate nucleic acids.) The sample is placed on a solid or semi-solid medium (e.g., a wet paper strip), electrodes are placed on each end of the medium, and an electrical current is passed from one electrode to the next. Each protein moves in a direction and at a rate that depends on its charge and its size.

**erythrocyte** (i-rith´rə-sīt), the hemoglobin-containing red cell in the blood.

**erythropoiesis** (i-rith-rō-poi-ē´sis), the process by which the stem cells in the bone marrow are converted into red cells.

**erythropoietin** (i-rith´rō-poi-ē´tin), a hormone that regulates the formation of erythrocytes from stem cells in the bone marrow. Often called EPO.

**GHb**, an unofficial, but often used, abbreviation for glycohemoglobin, a group of compounds formed when glucose in the blood attaches at one of several sites on the hemoglobin molecule.

**globin** (gl´bin), one of the proteins (i.e., long chains of amino acids) that combines with heme to form one heme-globin unit that is one-fourth of a hemoglobin molecule.

**haptoglobin** (hăp´-tə-gl-bin), a protein in the serum that aids in the removal of free hemoglobin from the blood.

**Hb**, a common, but not official, abbreviation for hemoglobin. The British often use Hgb.

**Hb A**, hemoglobin A – the major hemoglobin component of the greatest number of normal adults.

**Hb A$_2$**, a normal hemoglobin component present in adults at a concentration of 1.5-3%. It is elevated in beta-thalassemia.

**Hb F**, hemoglobin F – the major hemoglobin component of the fetus

**Hb S**, hemoglobin S – the hemoglobin variant responsible for sickle-cell anemia

**heme** (hmə), the flat, disk-shaped molecule containing iron that forms the non-protein portion of hemoglobin.

**hemoglobin** (h′mə-gl-bən), also spelled *haemoglobin*, the molecule in the red cells of the blood responsible for transporting oxygen.

**hemoglobinopathy** (hmə-gl-bən-op′ə-thē), a genetic disorder affecting the hemoglobin molecule either by reduced production of globins (a thalassemia) or by production of a hemoglobin variant that is a mutation of one of the normal hemoglobin components. Hb S, Hb E, and Hb G-Philadelphia are common hemoglobin variants.

**hemolysis** (hi-mŏl′i-sis), the rupturing of red cells.

**hemolyze** (h′mə-līz′), to rupture the membrane surrounding the red cell and release the hemoglobin molecules into solution.

**heterozygous** (hĕt′ə-rō-zī′gəs), having a different genetic code at corresponding sites on the maternal and paternal chromosomes.

**homozygous** (h́mō-zī́-gəs), having the same gene on both the maternal and the paternal chromosome.

**myoglobin** (mī́ə-glṓbin), the molecule that stores and transports oxygen inside cells. It consists of one heme and one globin chain.

**nucleotide** (nǘklē-ə-tīd́), one of the organic molecules that is used to form the genetic code in DNA and RNA (adenine, thymine, cytosine, guanine, and uracil).

**porphyria** (pôr-fîŕē-ə), a hereditary disorder related to the production of porphyrin (a precursor of heme) in the bone marrow or the liver.

**porphyrin** (pôŕfə-rin), a type of organic compound containing nitrogen atoms that forms the basis for several molecules important in living organisms: hemoglobin, chlorophyll, and several important enzymes.

**RNA, ribonucleic acid** (rī́bō-nǘklā́ik aśid), molecules similar in structure to DNA that help transfer the genetic code and translate it to the formation of proteins. Messenger RNA (mRNA) takes a copy of the DNA code to the ribosome. For each amino acid there is a transfer RNA (tRNA). It has an amino acid on one end and that acid's corresponding three-nucleotide DNA code on the other.

**thalassemia** (thaĺə-sḗmē-ə), a genetic disorder that results in the reduced production of a globin chain and, as a result, reduced levels of the hemoglobin molecules made from that chain. The different thalassemias are identified by indicating the specific globin affected: alpha-thalassemia, beta-thalassemia, delta-thalassemia, etc.

# ADDITIONAL READINGS

Those who wish to read in greater detail about the hemoglobin molecule should look at the most comprehensive text on the subject: *Hemoglobin: Molecular, Genetic and Clinical Aspects*, H. Franklin Bunn, MD, and Bernard G. Forget, MD., W.B. Saunders Company, Philadelphia, 1986. It is a very technical text and is not recommended for those who do not have a good scientific background.

Another good, but rather technical, book that was written for medical students and concentrates on genetics with particular reference to thalassemias and hemoglobinopathies is *The New Genetics and Clinical Practice*, D.J. Weatherall, Oxford University Press, Oxford, 1985. For a good introduction to the biochemical principles of genetics read the book *Molecular Design of Life* by Lubert Stryer, W.H. Freeman, New York, 1988. It is a very good presentation and often uses the hemoglobin molecule as a specific example, but the reader will need some background in chemistry to get full value from the book.

Those who wish to read more on the historical development of our knowledge of blood and hemoglobin will enjoy the following books and articles:

Conley, C. Lockard. "Sickle-Cell Anemia – The First Molecular Disease," in *Blood Pure and Eloquent*, M. M. Weintrobe (ed.). New York: McGraw-Hill, 1980.

Edsall, John T. "Blood and Hemoglobin: The Evolution of Knowledge of Functional Adaption in a Biochemical System. Part I: The Adaptation of Chemical Structure to Function in Hemoglobin," *Journal of the History of Biology* 5(2):205-257, Fall 1972.

Judson, Horace. *The Eighth Day of Creation, The Makers of the Revolution in Biology*. Simon and Schuster, New York, 1979.

Nuland, Sherwin. *Doctors: The Biography of Medicine.* (Chapters on Hippocrates, Galen, Vesalius, and Harvey.) New York: Alfred A. Knopf, 1988.

Rapson, Helen. *The Circulation of the Blood.* London: Frederick Muller Limited, 1982

Singer, Charles. *A Short History of Anatomy & Physiology from the Greeks to Harvey.* New York: Dover Publications, Inc., 1957.

Weatherall, D.J., "Toward an Understanding of the Molecular Biology of Some Common Inherited Anemias: The Story of Thalassemia," in *Blood Pure and Eloquent*, M. M. Weintrobe (ed.). New York: McGraw-Hill, 1980.

The book *Sickle Cell Anemia* by Anthony Cerami and Elsie Washington, The Third Press, New York, 1974, provides a good general review of this disorder. A similar type of nontechnical review of anemia in general will be found in Marilynn Larkin's *What You Can Do About Anemia*, Dell Publishing Company, New York, 1993.

Good introductions to the illness of George III and his role in the American Revolution will be found in the chapter "Mad George" in Vivian Green's *The Madness of Kings*, New York, St. Martin's Press, 1993 and in *The King Who Lost America, A Portrait of the Life and Times of George III* by Alan Loyd, Doubleday & Company, Inc., Garden City, NY, 1971. However, for a complete discussion of the role porphyria played in the royal houses of Stuart, Tudor, Hanover, and Brandenburg-Prussia, read *George III and the Mad-Business*, Ida Macalpine and Richard Hunter, Pimlico, London, 1991.

Finally, for a better understanding of genetic screening, DNA, and molecular biology, look at the following books:

Harsanyi, Zsolt and Richard Hutton. *Genetic Prophecy: Beyond the Double Helix*. New York: Rawson, Wade Publishers, 1981.

Shapiro, Robert. *The Human Blueprint: The Race to Unlock the Secrets of Our Genetic Script*. New York: St. Martin's Press, 1991.

Suzuki, David and Peter Knudtson. *Genethics*. Cambridge: Harvard University Press, 1990.

# INDEX

## A

abnormal hemoglobins, 4, 104, 117
Adair, 40, 41, 149
ALA, 77, 130, 133, 137, 138
al-Nofis, 28, 29, 147
alpha-thalassemia, 99, 100, 101, 102, 110, 113, 153, 160
alveolus, 59, 61, 62, 63, 157
amino acids, 2, 17, 41, 43, 44, 48, 50, 68, 71, 74, 75, 76, 80, 81, 83, 87, 103, 112, 113, 117, 123, 142, 149, 150, 151, 152, 158
anatomy, 7, 25, 26, 27, 29
anemia, 4, 5, 6, 7, 8, 9, 10, 11, 13, 14, 17, 18, 19, 66, 87, 88, 89, 90, 91, 92, 93, 94, 98, 100, 101, 102, 105, 107, 108, 109, 111, 132, 137, 139, 140, 143, 145, 146, 152, 154, 155, 162
aplastic, 90
arteries, 23, 25, 26, 29, 30, 62, 147, 148

## B

Bernard, 34, 112, 161
beta-thalassemia, 96, 97, 98, 99, 100, 103, 114, 115, 141, 143, 144, 152, 153, 159, 160
black people, 8, 154

blindness, 122, 128
blood glucose, 4, 119, 120, 121, 122, 123, 124, 125, 127, 154
blood stream, 21, 66, 68, 72, 78, 90, 118, 122, 143, 149, 150, 151
Bohr, ix, x, 35, 53, 63, 64, 65, 66, 148
Bohr curve, 63, 64, 65, 66
Bradford, 94
Braunitzer, 48

## C

Caminoptros, 94
capillaries, 9, 14, 23, 25, 26, 29, 30, 32, 35, 36, 53, 62, 63, 64, 65, 80, 106, 147, 153
carbon dioxide, 2, 3, 21, 30, 31, 32, 35, 55, 56, 57, 59, 61, 62, 63, 65, 119, 130, 148, 150
Castle, 11, 12, 88
Cesalpino, 29, 30, 147
chlorophyll, 34, 42, 43, 148, 160
chromosome 11, 77, 82, 83, 96, 151
chromosome 16, 74, 77, 82, 99, 151
circulation, 22, 23, 27, 28, 29, 30, 66, 128, 142, 147, 154
Colombo, 29, 30, 147
Conant, 36, 37, 149
coronary thrombosis, 7

## D

deletion, 96, 102, 153
diabetes, 4, 119, 120, 121, 122, 124, 125, 126, 127, 128, 154
diabetics, xiv, 20, 119, 120, 121, 122, 123, 125, 127, 128, 154
Diggs, 8, 11
DNA, x, 18, 73, 74, 75, 76, 77, 81, 82, 89, 95, 96, 97, 99, 100, 112, 113, 114, 118, 130, 137, 138, 144, 147, 151, 153, 158, 160, 163

## E

electrophoresis, 12, 123, 124, 158
endocrine glands, 21, 23
Erasistratus, 25
erythropoietin, 73, 151, 158
excess water, 21

## F

Fischer, 7, 42

## G

G-6-PD deficiency, 91, 92, 152
Galen, 26, 27, 28, 29, 162
genes, 1, 4, 13, 14, 15, 17, 81, 94, 96, 98, 99, 100, 101, 103, 108, 110, 112, 114, 117, 137, 153
genetic disorders, 4, 94, 117, 134, 142, 146, 147, 154, 155
genetic information, 2, 17, 18, 81, 82, 95, 145, 151
George III, vii, 129, 134, 135, 136, 155, 162
GHb, xiv, 118, 119, 122, 123, 126, 127, 128, 154, 158
GHb test, 119, 122, 127
Gillespie, 9
Gipson, 132
glucose, 4, 65, 89, 118, 119, 120, 121, 122, 124, 125, 126, 127, 154, 158

glycohemoglobins, 4, 19, 126, 154
Guthrie, 141

## H

Hahn, 9
Harvey, 12, 13, 30, 66, 147, 162
Hasselbach, 35, 65, 148
Hb A, x, 11, 14, 17, 66, 82, 83, 93, 95, 96, 97, 99, 102, 104, 106, 108, 110, 123, 124, 125, 126, 127, 128, 151, 152, 159
Hb A$_{1c}$, 124, 125, 126, 127
Hb A$_2$, 83, 93, 95, 96, 97, 99, 106, 123, 151, 152, 159
Hb C, 109, 112, 113
Hb Constant Springs, 112
Hb D, 110
Hb E, 109, 115, 154, 159
Hb F, 3, 11, 14, 66, 83, 93, 98, 104, 106, 108, 117, 143, 144, 151, 152, 155, 159
Hb G-Philadelphia, 104, 110, 111, 159
Hb H disease, 101, 102, 113, 153
Hb Köln, 111
Hb Lepore, x, 113, 114, 115
Hb M, 104, 111, 112
Hb S, x, 14, 17, 76, 90, 95, 105, 106, 107, 108, 109, 110, 115, 123, 127, 143, 153, 154, 155, 159
heart, 6, 9, 22, 23, 25, 26, 27, 28, 29, 30, 59, 87, 98, 122
Heinz bodies, 80
heme, 2, 33, 34, 39, 41, 42, 43, 48, 50, 51, 52, 53, 62, 68, 71, 77, 78, 79, 80, 81, 82, 88, 129, 130, 131, 133, 134, 136, 137, 138, 149, 150, 151, 154, 158, 159, 160
hemoglobinopathy, 90, 105, 117, 146, 159
hemoglobins, 12, 13, 14, 69, 81, 82, 102, 117, 118, 124, 128, 150, 151, 154
hemolytic, 7, 90, 91, 92, 152
Henry, 31, 36, 135
Herophilis, 25
Herrick, 5, 6, 7
Hill, 7, 48
Hippocrates, 24, 162

Hoppe-Seyler, 33, 34, 42, 85, 148
hormones, 21, 23
Howell-Jolly bodies, 79, 80
Hüfner, ix, 35, 63, 148
Hunter, 134, 136, 163
hydrops fetalis, 101, 102, 110, 153

## I

Ingram, 17, 48, 95
insulin, 119, 120, 121, 122, 128
iron, 2, 36, 37, 39, 40, 41, 42, 43, 51, 52,
    53, 61, 62, 66, 68, 71, 78, 80, 87, 89,
    92, 98, 111, 130, 131, 133, 148, 149,
    150, 152, 159
Itano, 12, 13, 14

## J

James I, 134, 135

## K

Kendrew, 49
kidneys, 6, 21, 23, 68, 69, 73, 90, 91, 122,
    128, 132, 150
Konigsberg, 48
Krogh, 35, 148
Kunkel, 95
Kuster, 42

## L

Landsteiner, 68
Lavoisier, 30, 148
lead poisoning, 4, 131, 132, 133, 154
Lee, 94
Linus Pauling, 11, 12, 13, 123
liver, 6, 23, 25, 26, 68, 80, 81, 88, 89, 92,
    94, 98, 119, 129, 132, 160
lungs, 2, 3, 6, 9, 21, 22, 25, 26, 28, 29, 30,
    32, 35, 36, 53, 56, 57, 59, 60, 63, 65,
    133, 148, 149, 150

## M

Macalpine, 134, 136, 163
macrophages, 80, 151
malaria, 10, 11, 92
Malpighi, 30
Minot, 88
mRNA, 75, 76, 96, 97, 99, 100, 112, 113,
    138, 151, 160
Murphy, 88
myoglobin, 35, 49, 53, 62, 63, 64, 129,
    148, 149, 150, 160

## N

nerves, 122
nitrogen, 31, 39, 42, 44, 51, 57, 59, 77, 79,
    149, 160
Nixon, 4, 18, 19, 139
normoblast, 73, 74, 77, 78
nucleotides, 73, 151, 158
nutritional diseases, 5

## O

osmotic pressure, 40, 41, 149
oxygen, 2, 3, 7, 8, 9, 11, 12, 14, 21, 22, 23,
    30, 31, 32, 34, 35, 36, 37, 39, 44, 49,
    50, 51, 52, 53, 55, 56, 57, 59, 60, 61,
    62, 63, 64, 65, 66, 67, 68, 69, 73, 87,
    90, 93, 96, 98, 101, 102, 105, 106, 107,
    111, 112, 129, 140, 148, 149, 150, 152,
    153, 154, 159, 160

## P

pain, 4, 6, 7, 8, 9, 106, 107, 122, 134, 135,
    140, 144, 154, 155
pancreas, 99, 119, 120
Patricelli, 18
Pauling, 11, 12, 13, 14, 17, 18, 48, 104,
    112
pernicious, 11, 88, 89
Perutz, 49, 50, 52, 149
PKU, 141, 142, 143

porphyrin, 42, 51, 52, 78, 79, 130, 149, 160
porphyrins, 42, 43, 134, 149
pronormoblast, 73
protein, 1, 2, 3, 5, 7, 13, 17, 18, 19, 33, 39, 41, 43, 44, 48, 50, 53, 69, 74, 75, 76, 77, 89, 95, 96, 97, 112, 113, 130, 138, 147, 148, 149, 151, 158, 159
protein synthesis, 147
pyrolle, 42, 43, 79
Pythagoras, 90, 91, 153

## R

red blood cells, 10, 21, 68, 73, 87, 91
respiration, xiii, xiv, 3, 5, 19, 30, 42, 147, 148
respiratory pigments, 57
reticulocyte, 78
reticulum, 71, 72
Rhinesmith, 48
RNA, x, 74, 75, 76, 95, 96, 97, 138, 147, 151, 157, 160

## S

Schroeder, 48
Servetus, 27, 28, 29, 147
Sherman, 9
sickle-cell, 5, 6, 7, 8, 9, 10, 11, 12, 13, 14, 15, 16, 17, 18, 19, 76, 90, 94, 96, 97, 98, 103, 104, 105, 106, 107, 108, 109, 127, 139, 140, 141, 142, 143, 144, 145, 146, 153, 154, 155, 159
sickle-cell anemia, 5, 6, 7, 8, 9, 10, 11, 12, 13, 14, 15, 16, 17, 18, 19, 76, 96, 97, 98, 103, 104, 105, 106, 107, 108, 109, 139, 140, 141, 143, 144, 145, 146, 153, 154, 155, 159
siderotic granules, 80

spleen, 25, 68, 79, 80, 94, 98, 145, 146, 151
stem cells, 144, 150, 152, 158
Stokes, 34, 35, 148
Stretton, 95
swelling, 9, 106
Sydenstrucker, 8

## T

Teichman, 32, 39
thalassemia, 90, 93, 94, 95, 96, 115, 117, 159, 160
tRNA, 75, 76, 151, 160
Turner, 132

## V

Van Neel, 14
veins, 11, 23, 24, 25, 26, 29, 30, 59, 63, 147, 148
Vesalius, 27, 29, 162
vision, 6, 122, 128, 154
vitamin $B_{12}$, 87, 88, 89, 152

## W

Wallenius, 95
waste products, 21, 23
Wells, 13, 14
Whipple, 94
WIC, 85, 89

## Z

Zinoffsky, 39
ZnPP, 133